TAOIST CHI KUNG

STRATEGIES

LEVEL 1 | Jing · *Essence*

LEVEL 2 | Chi · *Energy*

LEVEL 3 | Shen · *Spirit*

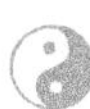

Larry Johnson | O.M.D.,L.AC.

WHITE ELEPHANT MONASTERY PRESS

TAOIST CHI KUNG

STRATEGIES

COPYRIGHT © 2026 Larry Johnson

All rights reserved. No part of this book may be reproduced or transmitted in any form or by any means, electronic or mechanical, including photocopying, recording, or by any information storage and retrieval system, without permission in writing from the publisher.

THIRD EDITION

ISBN 979-8-9892335-9-5

DESIGN · Curt Carpenter

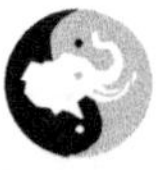

White Elephant Monastery Press
PO Box 787
Crestone, Colorado 81131

*Note to the Reader
and a Disclaimer*

The information in this book is presented for educational and entertainment purposes only.

All therapies, treatments, diagnosis, exercises and physical or energetic interventions of any and all natures should be undertaken only under the direct guidance and care of a properly trained and legally licensed health care professional specializing in the techniques and services rendered.

Nothing described in this book should be construed by any reader or other person to be a diagnosis or treatment for any disease or condition and neither the author, publisher, nor any distributors can accept responsibility for any ill effects resulting from the use or misuse of the information contained herein.

Any use or misuse of the information presented here for educational and entertainment purposes is the sole responsibility of the reader.

Any such use or misuse is at his or her own risk.

TAOIST CHI KUNG
STRATEGIES

TABLE OF CONTENTS

Introduction

IN APRIL OF 1976, I was introduced to Chan Chiu Lim by Sam Louie, a prominent Choy Lee Fut Kung Fu practitioner and one of Sifu Chans' few Chi Kung students. I had been hearing about Sifu Chan through the Chinese Martial Arts grapevine in San Francisco for some time. He was reported to be the master of a very ancient Taoist System of Chi Kung. Both Sifu Chan, who was to become my teacher for the next twenty five years, and his system were elusive. I was fortunate enough to be part of the Choy Lee Fut Martial Arts community, and through that association prevailed upon Sam to call Sifu Chan and ask him to meet me. At that first meeting Sifu Chan accepted me as a student, thus beginning my wondrous journey of a serious study of Taoist Chi Kung.

Our system has been shrouded in secrecy for hundreds, if not thousands, of years. At my first lesson, Sifu Chan asked me to keep my training secret, a request I honored for many years. Later, when I was given permission to teach the system, Sifu was rather insistent that I did pass on what I had learned.

This book is not an instruction manual for Taoist Chi Kung. It would be foolish for anyone to attempt to learn this sophisticated art without personal attention from a qualified teacher. Our version of a qualified teacher is one who has practiced several hours a day for a minimum of eight years and has permission to teach.

The real purpose of this book is to tell a story. The process of Spiritual/Energetic development has been understood since ancient times. Many traditions have documented complete, step by step approaches to self realization. The emphasis here is on "complete, step by step." Each of these documentations is a "story" containing a clear beginning, and an orderly progression to the end.

With the explosion of communication technology in the world today, enormous amounts of information are being disseminated, not always accurately and not always completely accurately and not always completely. Pieces of various "stories" are circulating around, often being misinterpreted as complete. Sometimes different "stories" have been combined to form new tales which do not necessarily contain the richness from which their parts were drawn.

Problems can arise when incomplete, superficially fabricated, or out of order "stories" are matriculated into the weave of our lives. At best they will not serve and at worst may damage.

The goal of *Strategies* is to convey the complete story as told by one ancient tradition. It is certainly not represented as the only story, but it is one that has remained intact through the ages.

May this story be entertaining, educational, and thought provoking. ☯

—LARRY JOHNSON

CHAPTER 1

Background

CHI

CHI IS DEFINED as vital energy—in the large sense the "stuff" underlying all manifestation in the universe. Chi inside the human body is both a carrier and a message. It transfers both energy and information. Chi emitted from a Chi Kung Master contains infrared radiation, particle streams, static electricity, etc.

There are two general classifications of Chi inside the body, Prenatal and Postnatal.

Prenatal Chi (Source Chi) refers to the vital energy given to the human at birth from both parents. It is the basic matter (Essence) and native force that support the body's tissues and organs. This Chi is directly related to Ming Men and the Eight Extra-Ordinary Vessels of the body *(see pg. 14 & 15)*.

Postnatal Chi is a combination of Chi derived from the food we eat and the air we breath that sustains our vital functions. This Chi is directly related to the 12 Primary Meridian/Organ Systems of the body.

Together the Prenatal and Postnatal Chi form the True Chi of the body. True Chi is the source of energy used in daily life.

Chi Kung was developed to balance, harmonize, and enhance the True Chi for health and longevity and to transform the True Chi for Spiritual Development. Chi Kung exercises can also directly impact Prenatal Chi, Postnatal Chi, Essence, and Spirit—that which directs our life activities and links us to the Divine.

YIN AND YANG

YIN AND YANG are the two opposing, yet interdependent and complementary aspects of all existence. They can be used to describe the relationships between the qualities of all things. Imbalances in any one or more of the Yin/Yang aspects of our being results in illness. Yin/Yang balance on the other hand promotes wellness.

The basic properties of Yang are likened to fire and the basic properties of Yin are likened to water. Yang qualities are hot, bright, rising, expanding, daytime, Spring, Summer, external, etc. In the human body Yang relates to the top, back, left side, and exterior. The bowels are considered Yang inside the body and Heaven is Yang outside the body.

Yin qualities are cold, dim, sinking, contracting, nighttime, Fall, Winter, internal, etc. In the human body Yin relates to the bottom, front, right side, and interior. The viscera are considered Yin inside the body and Earth is Yin outside the body.

Because Yin and Yang are so closely connected and interdependent, any imbalance in one of them will soon affect the other. They are involved in a constantly changing energetic play called life. The play is staged within certain limits called balance. When these limits are breached by either Yin or Yang, there is sickness. Death, signifying the total divorce of the Yin/Yang relationship, is the end of the play.

THE 12 MAJOR ORGANS/MERIDIANS

ACCORDING TO CHI KUNG THEORY, the human body is nourished, protected and balanced by a complex network of Chi transporting channels. From each single cell to all the tissues and organs of the body, it is these channels which maintain and support the process of life. There are several classifications of these channels including Primary Meridians, Luo-Connecting

Channels, Divergent Channels, Extra-Ordinary Channels, Sinen Channels, and Minute Channels. Each has its sphere of influence and function in maintaining the health of our body/mind complex.

A study of the channel system for the Chi Kung student is much like studying anatomy for the medical student. Such an in-depth study is far beyond the scope of this book. There are numerous publications on the market that can do justice to this subject.

For the purposes of this book we will confine ourselves to addressing the Twelve Primary Meridians and the Eight Extra-Ordinary Vessels. When we look at an acupuncture chart, it is usually the Twelve Primary Meridians with their associated points that are depicted. The Twelve Meridians run vertically and bi-laterally on the body, each connecting with an organ (or function in the case of the Pericardium and Triple Heater) but influencing a much larger orb in the body than the area directly covered by the meridian.

Six meridians flow through the arms and six meridians flow through the legs. The Pericardium, Heart, and Lung Meridians are Yin and flow through the inner surface of the arm from chest to hand. The Triple Heater, Small Intestine, and Large Intestine Meridians are Yang and flow through the outer surface of the arm from hand to head. The Gall Bladder, Urinary Bladder, and Stomach are Yang Meridians that flow from the head down the body and along the outer surface of the leg to the feet while the Liver, Kidney, and Spleen are Yin Meridians that flow from the feet along the inner surface of the legs to the chest.

The Meridians are grouped into Yin/Yang pairs with the Yin Meridians being considered internal and the Yang Meridians being considered external.

The Meridians circulate vital energy and blood, warm and nourish the tissues, and link and support the various structural and functional aspects of the whole being while providing the route for internal man to communicate with the cosmos.

Each meridian has specific locations where the deeper energies of the body may be accessed from the outside. These locations are called acupuncture points. Each point acts on the body's energy in a specific manner. This is called the function of the point. The functions vary from point to point, and from point combination to point combination. In other words, the function of a point can be altered depending on which other points are being stimulated at the same time.

YANG ORGANS

THE MAIN FUNCTIONS of the Yang Organs are to receive and digest food, to absorb nutrients and to excrete waste material.

The Gall Bladder forms a Yin/Yang pair with the Liver. Its main function is to store bile and secrete it into the Small Intestine to aid digestion. It is the only Yang organ that stores a pure liquid (bile).

The Stomach forms a Yin/Yang pair with the Spleen. Its main functions are to receive and decompose food, temporarily store it, and pass it to the Small Intestine for further digestion.

The Small Intestine forms a Yin/Yang pair with the Heart. Its main functions are to receive partially digested food from the Stomach, temporarily store it while assimilating nutrients, and pass the residue to the Large Intestine.

The Large Intestine is Yin/Yang paired with the Lung. Its main functions are to receive waste from the Small Intestine, absorb part of the liquid, turn the rest to feces, and transport the feces to the anus for excretion.

The Urinary Bladder is Yin/Yang paired with the Kidneys. Its main functions are to temporarily store urine and discharge it when the proper amount is in storage.

The Triple Burner is Yin/Yang paired with the Pericardium. Both are functions rather than physical organs. Although the Triple Burner is classified as a Yang organ, it is really the combination of the physiological activities of three areas of the body:

- The Upper Burner is the chest area and generalizes the functions of the Lung and Heart in transporting blood and vital energy throughout the body.

- The Middle Burner is the epigastric area and generalizes the functions of the Spleen and Stomach in digesting food and absorbing nutrients.

- The Lower Burner is the hypogastric area and generalizes the functions of the Urinary Bladder and Kidneys in controlling water metabolism. It is also the residence of our Prenatal or Source Chi which is our inherited constitutional energy.

YIN ORGANS

THE MAIN FUNCTIONS of the Yin organs are to manufacture and store essential substances such as Chi, Essence, and body fluids.

The Liver is Yin/Yang paired with the Gall Bladder. Its main functions are to store blood, nourish the tendons, and maintain the smooth flow of Chi throughout the body.

The Heart is Yin/Yang paired with the Small Intestine and is considered the overall ruler of the body, home of Shen (the controlling Spirit of the body/mind complex). Its main functions are to control the blood vessels and house the mind.

The Spleen (including the Pancreas) is Yin/Yang paired with the Stomach. Its main functions are to govern digestion, absorption, and transmission of nutrients to the body, keep the blood in the vessels, hold the organs in place, and nourish the muscles. It is also involved in water metabolism.

The Lungs are Yin/Yang paired with the Large Intestine. The main functions of the Lungs are to control respiration, regulate the water passages and nourish the skin and hair. Regulating the water passages refers to the functions of turning part of the body fluid into sweat to be excreted through the pores in the skin, controlling the pores, and sending part of the body fluid down to the Kidney/Urinary Bladder complex.

The Kidney is Yin/Yang paired with the Urinary Bladder. Its main functions are to store essential substances, dominate reproduction, growth, and development, produce marrow, control bones and receive air from the Lungs.

The Pericardium is Yin/Yang related to the Triple Burner. Its main functions are to protect the Heart and to relay orders from the Heart to the rest of the body.

FIVE ELEMENTS—PHASES

THE FIVE ELEMENTS, wood, fire, earth, metal, and water, are symbols for natural processes inherent in all things. They provide a pattern of change in which all phenomena can be classified including the physiology and pathology of the organs, tissues, and emotions of humans.

Five Element Correspondences

	Wood	*Fire*	*Earth*	*Metal*	*Water*
Viscera	liver	heart	spleen	lung	kidney
Bowel	gall bladder	small intestine	stomach	large intestine	urinary bladder
Color	green	red	yellow	white	black/blue
Emotion	anger	joy	reminiscence	grief/sorrow	fear/fright
Tissue	tendon	blood vessels	muscle	skin/sense	bone
Sense Organ	eyes	tongue	mouth	nose	ears
Season	sping	summer	late summer	fall	winter
Taste	sour	bitter	sweet	pungent	salty
Direction	east	south	middle	west	north
Climate	wind	heat	damp	dry	cold
Nature	birth	growth	mature	harvest	store
Sound	shout	laugh	sing	weep	groan
Liquid Emitted	tears	sweat	saliva	mucous	urine
Grain	wheat	millet	rye	rice	beans
Meat	chicken	mutton	beef	horse	pork
Nourishes	nails	complexion	lips	body hair	head hair

THERE ARE THIRTY six possible interacting relationships or cycles for the Five Elements. The most important cycles are the promoting, controlling, over-acting, and counter-acting.

Promoting personifies the "mother-son" principle of Chinese Medicine. Each element promotes—is the mother of—one element and is promoted by—is the son of—another. Thus Wood promotes Fire, Fire promotes Earth, Earth promotes Metal, Metal promotes Water and Water promotes Wood.

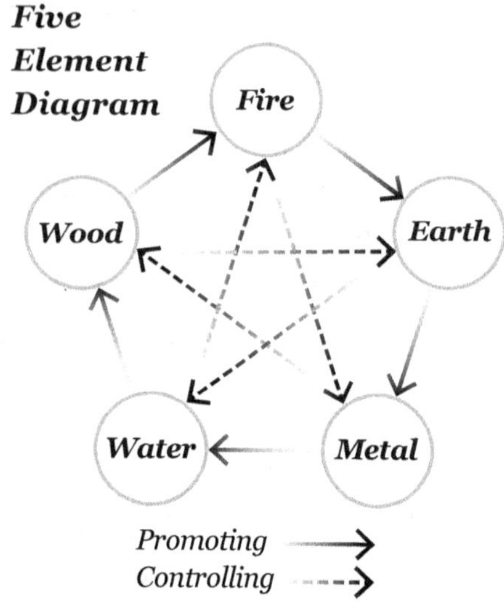

In the controlling cycle, Wood controls Earth, Earth controls Water, Water controls Fire, Fire controls Metal, and Metal controls Wood. Both the promoting and controlling cycles are necessary for proper balance.

Over-acting and counter-acting cycles occur when one of the Elements is in a state of either deficiency or excess, and often they appear together. Over-acting follows the same pathway as the control cycle. For instance if Wood was in excess it could overact on Earth, or if Water was deficient Earth could over-act on it. The counter-acting cycle follows the reverse pathway of the control cycle. If Wood was in excess it could counter-act on Metal or if Metal was deficient Wood could counteract on it.

When any internal organ is in a state of imbalance it can directly affect its son, mother, the organ it controls, and the organ that controls it.

THE TWELVE MAJOR ORGANS/MERIDIANS

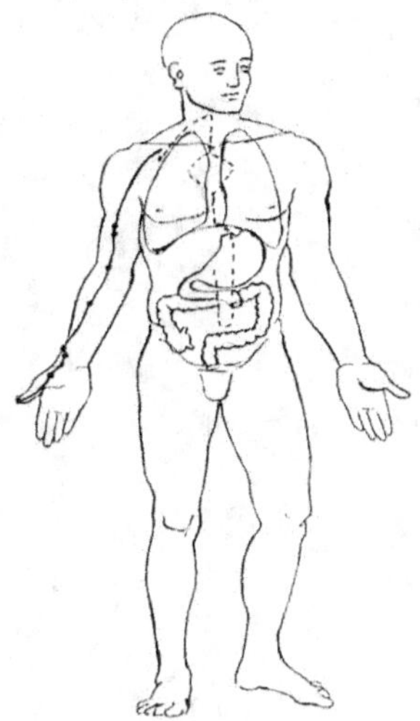

Lung Channel

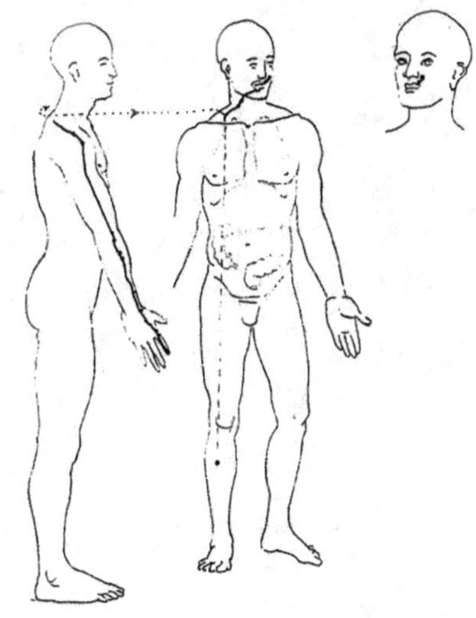

Large Intestine Channel

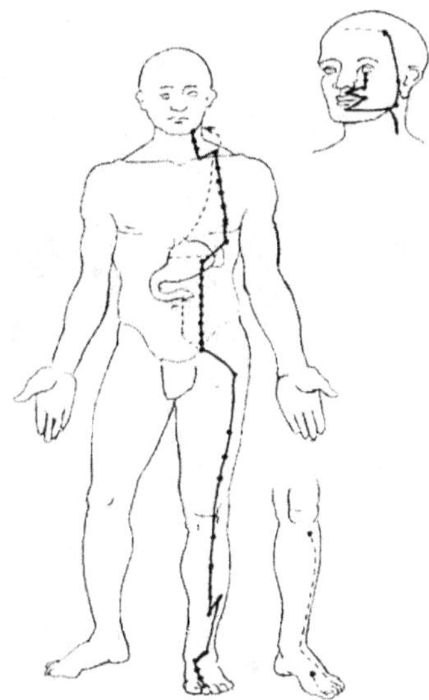

Stomach Channel

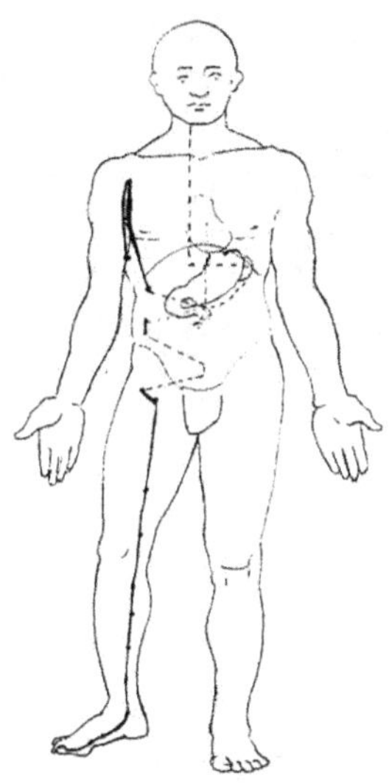

Spleen Channel

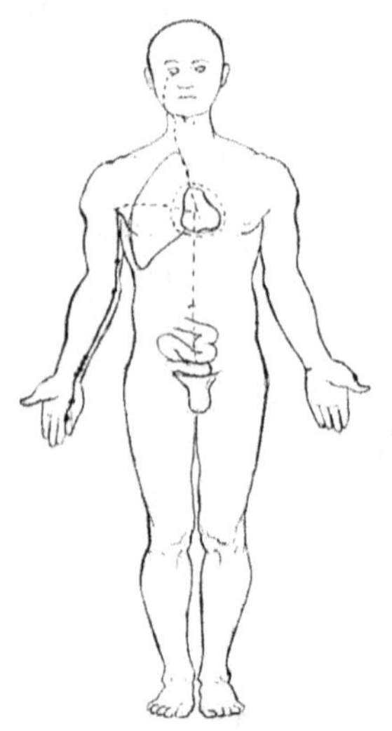

Heart Channel

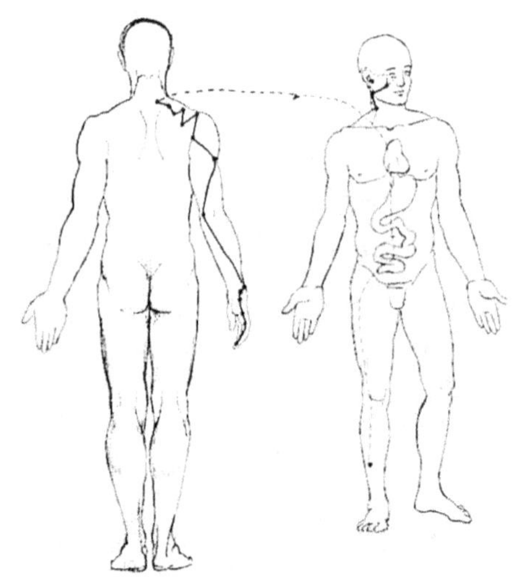

Small Intestine Channel

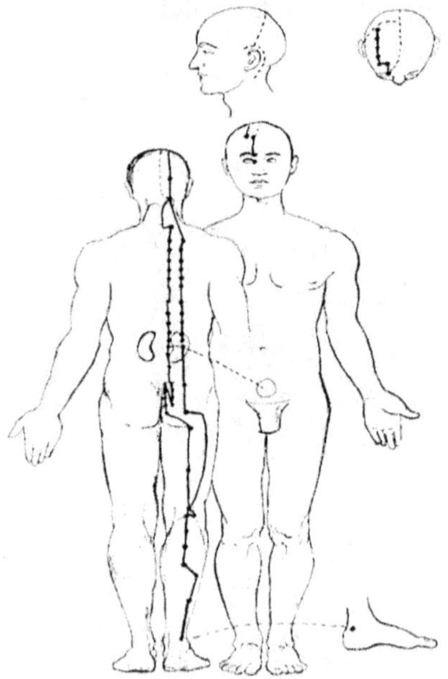

Urinary Bladder Channel

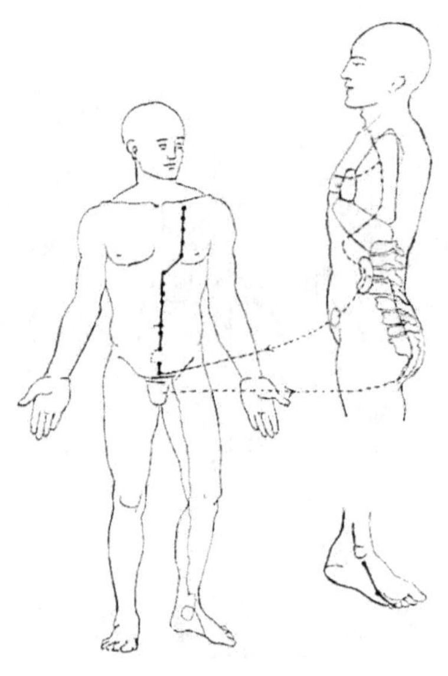

Kidney Channel

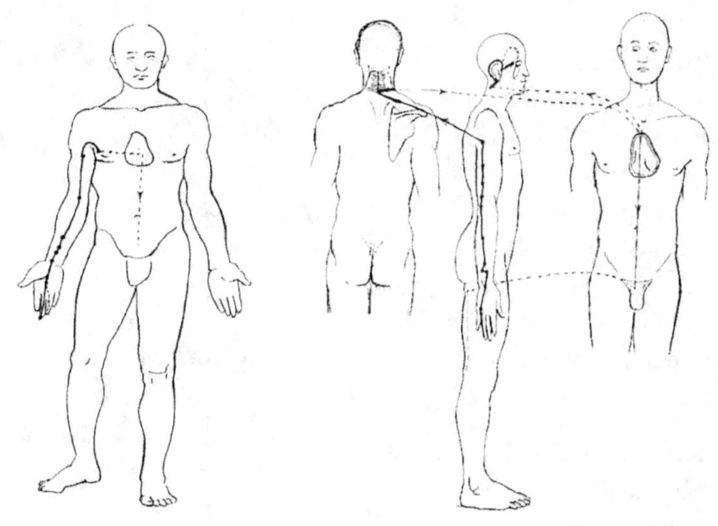

Pericardium Channel   Triple Burner Channel

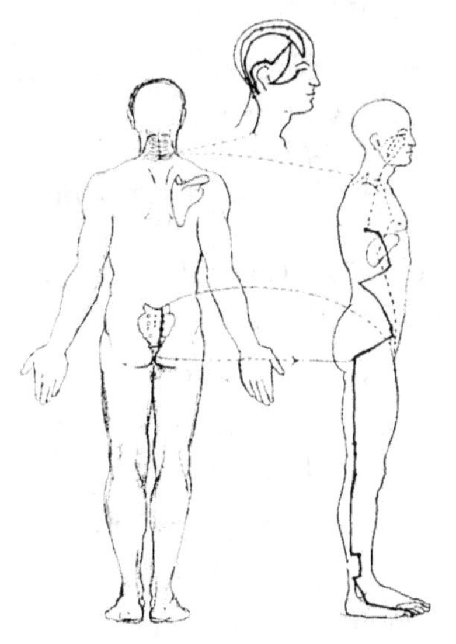

Gall Bladder Channel

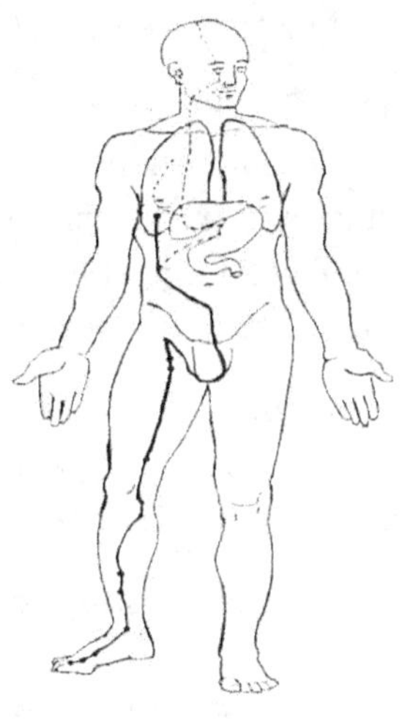

Liver Channel

MING MEN is the first and most important energy center in the body. First because it is formed at the moment of conception before the fetus is formed and most important because it is the center of energetic transformations.

Bi-lateral Ming Men, located in the Kidneys, has seven energy channels connecting it's two sides called the Moving Chi between the Kidneys. Ming Men is where Heaven and Earth meet in man and interact to produce life.

Prenatal Chi, Postnatal Chi and cosmic energy interface and transform in

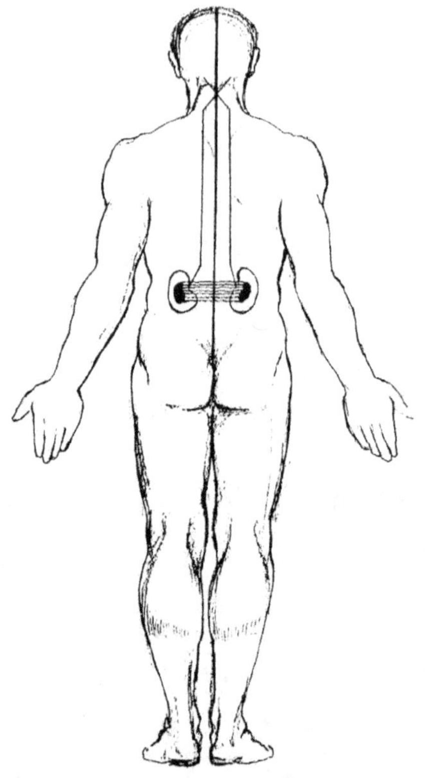

Ming Men

Ming Men to support life. It is the origin of the Governing Vessel, the Conception Vessel, Chong Mai and the Triple Heater.

The Governing Vessel and the Conception Vessel are often considered the Yang and Yin branches of the Moving Chi between the Kidneys. Source Chi and Spirit are stored in the Ming Men.

Ming Men itself is often considered the back of the Lower Tan Tien. In fact, the Lower Tan Tien, Moving Chi between the Kidneys and Ming Men are so intimately connected that they can be considered one.

THE EIGHT EXTRA-ORDINARY VESSELS

THE EIGHT Extra-Ordinary Vessels have a deep relationship with the inseparable structure/energy complex of the body and the exchange of information throughout the body.

At the first division of the fertilized egg the Governing and Conception Vessels are formed and at the second division the Belt Channel emerges. A child in the womb relies on the Eight Extra-Ordinary Vessels for all its body functions while the other channels of its body are being developed.

After birth, the Twelve Primary Meridians maintain life function while the Extra-Ordinary Vessels help regulate the Twelve Primary Meridians. The Extra-Ordinary Vessels act as reservoirs of Chi and Blood in the body, absorbing excess and repleting deficiency. They have direct relationships with the brain and spinal cord, hormonal control, the skeletal system, the genitalia, the circulatory system, the production of blood and the hepatic and biliary systems. Their influence on our body/mind/Spirit complex is deep and profound.

Each Extra-Ordinary Vessel has a bi-lateral Acupuncture point (Master Point) that controls it.

DU MAI
GOVERNING VESSEL

THE GOVERNING Vessel, known as the Sea of Yang, helps regulate all the Yang of the body and through the acupuncture point GV 14 links all the Yang Channels. Du Mai controls the dorsal aspect of the body. The acupuncture point that controls Du Mai is Small Intestine 3.

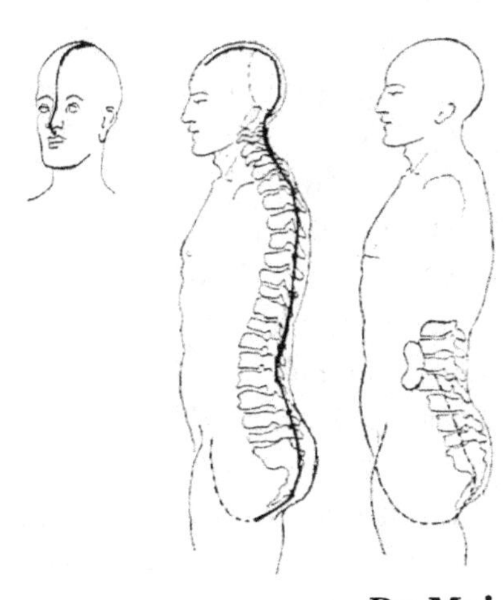

Du Mai
Governing Vessel

REN MAI
CONCEPTION VESSEL

THE CONCEPTION VESSEL, known as the Sea of Yin, helps regulate all the Yin in the body and links all the Yin channels. Ren Mai controls the ventral aspect of the body. The acupuncture point that controls Ren Mai is Lung 7.

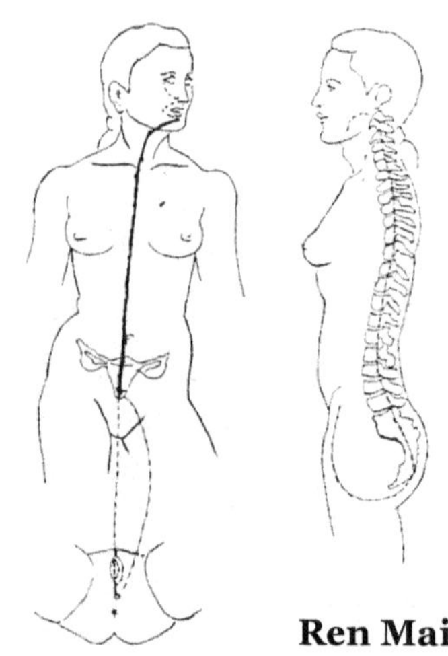

Ren Mai
Conception Vessel

CHONG MAI
VITALITY VESSEL

CHONG MAI, known as the Sea of Blood and the Sea of the Twelve Meridians, is the main purveyor of Source Chi in the body. It strengthens the link between the Conception and Governing Vessels and is said to regulate the sinens and meridians of the whole body. The upper part of Chong

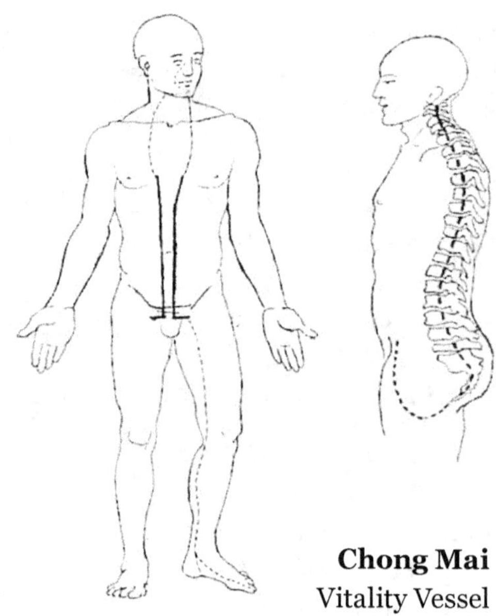

Chong Mai
Vitality Vessel

Mai connects with all the Yang Meridians and the lower part connects with all the Yin meridians. The acupuncture point that controls Chong Mai is Spleen 4.

DAI MAI
BELT VESSEL

THE BELT CHANNEL circles the waist linking all the vertical channels on the abdomen. It has an especially close and binding relationship with the Conception Vessel, Chong Mai, Gall Bladder, Liver, Spleen, and Kidney Meridians. The Belt Channel gets energy from the Liver and Gall Bladder Meridians and receives Source Chi from the Kidneys. The Chi Kung community recognizes its direct connection with Ming Men although this is not mentioned often in the Chinese Medical community. By regulating the vertical channels on the abdomen, the Belt Channel harmonizes energy between the upper and lower parts of the body. The acupuncture point that controls Dai Mai is Gall Bladder 41.

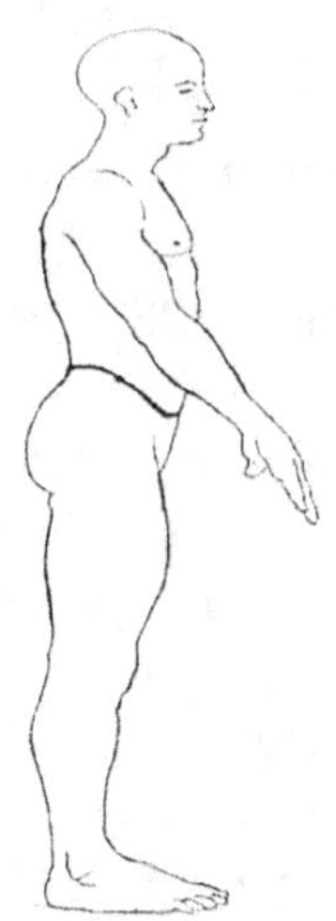

Dai Mai
Belt Vessel

YANG CHIAO MAI
YANG HEEL VESSEL

THE YANG HEEL CHANNEL links the Urinary Bladder, Gall Bladder, Small Intestine, Large Intestine, and Stomach Channels. It is somewhat regarded as a branch of the Urinary Bladder Meridian. The Yang Heel Channel controls the amount and movement of Yang energy in the body, dominates activity and corresponds to the energy of Heaven. The acupuncture point that controls Yang Chiao Mai is Urinary Bladder 62.

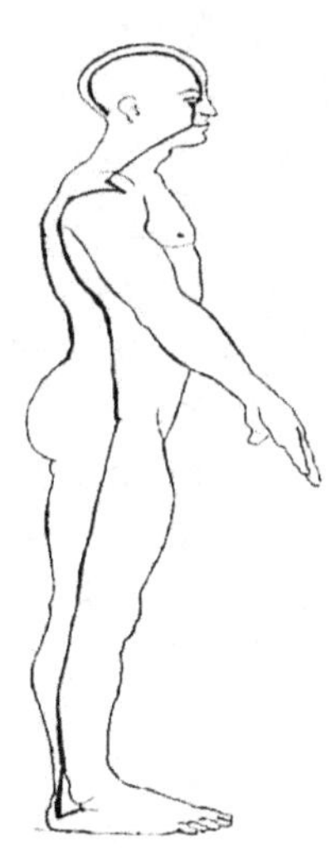

Yang Chiao Mai
Yang Heel Vessel

YIN CHIAO MAI
YIN HEEL VESSEL

THE YIN HEEL CHANNEL links the Kidney and Urinary Bladder Channels and is somewhat regarded as a secondary branch of the Kidney Meridian. It controls the amount of and movement of Yin in the body, dominates quietness, and corresponds to the energy of Earth. The acupuncture point that controls Yin Chiao Mai is Kidney 6.

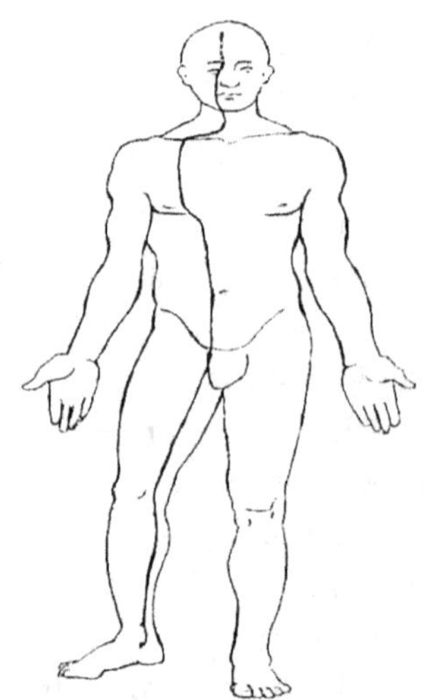

Yin Chiao Mai
Yin Heel Vessel

YIN WEI MAI
YIN LINKING VESSEL

THE YIN LINKING CHANNEL dominates the interior of the body, with an especially powerful effect on the Conception Vessel, Heart and Lung. It also connects with the Kidney, Spleen, and Liver. Like the Chong Mai it contains Source Chi. It is mainly concerned with regulating the deep energies of the body. The acupuncture point that controls the Yin Wei Mai is Pericardium 6.

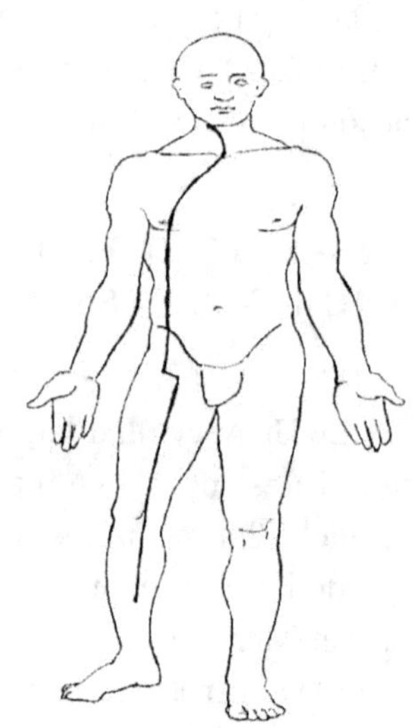

Yin Wei Mai
Yin Linking Vessel

YANG WEI MAI
YANG LINKING VESSEL

THE YANG LINKING CHAN-NEL dominates the exterior of
the body, connecting with the Triple
Heater, Gall Bladder, Urinary Bladder,
Small Intestine, Stomach, and Gov-erning Vessel. It is mainly concerned
with regulating the defensive energy
of the body. The acupuncture point
that controls Yang Wei Mai is Triple
Heater 5.

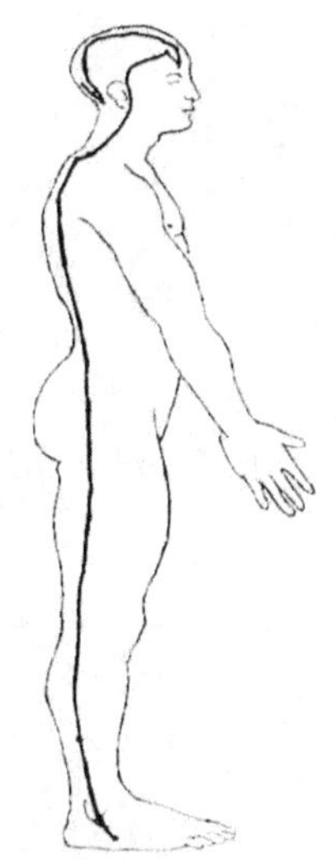

Yang Wei Mai
Yang Linking Vessel

EACH EXTRA-ORDINARY Vessel has a bilateral Master
Point (as mentioned above) on one of the limbs that
activates it. The Vessels have their own functions and can be
used therapeutically alone, but they have been shown to work
very effectively in specific pairs. The paired Vessels support and
augment the functions of each other. Dai Mai works with Yang Wei
Mai—Du Mai works with Yang Chaio Mai—Chong Mai works with
Yin Wei Mai—Ren Mai works with Yin Chaio Mai. The Master
Point of one of each pair is on the upper limb and the Master Point
of the other member of the pair is on the lower limb.

THE EIGHT EXTRA-ORDINARY VESSELS

ARE THE PATHWAYS

OF SPIRITUAL TRANSFORMATION

CHAPTER 2

Chi Kung

*Chi Kung requires that the practitioner regulate the body,
breath and mind.
Body position is the base, breath is the activator
and mind is the guide.*

THERE ARE TWO BASIC TYPES OF CHI KUNG—QUIET AND MOVING.

QUIET OR STATIC Chi Kung can be performed while standing, sitting or lying as long as there is no body movement. The emphasis in this type is usually on the internal organs and energy systems and utilizes the body shape and mind to move the Chi. The goal here is movement in stillness. The cerebral cortex remains relatively still in Quiet Chi Kung. Some Quiet Chi Kung positions are quite strenuous and also exercise the muscles, tendons and bones.

Moving or Dynamic Chi Kung requires movement of the trunk or limbs. This causes more excitement of the cerebral cortex. The goal here is to be externally active but internally still. Body shape, motion and the mind are used to move the Chi. In Moving Chi Kung, the internal energy systems and organs are developed as well as the muscles, tendons and bones.

1 | REGULATING BREATH

BREATH REGULATION requires the control of the quantity, quality, duration and destination of the breath. Generally speaking Chi Kung requires your breathing to be of long duration on both the inhale and the exhale. A much larger amount of air is inhaled and exhaled than usual and the breath is qualitatively very soft. The destination is dependent on the specific exercise being performed. In some exercises these parameters change for specific reasons.

Breath regulation increases the efficiency of the oxygen/carbon dioxide exchange. This ensures the whole body and especially the brain has an abundant supply of oxygen and that waste materials are removed expediently. This in itself constitutes an inner cleansing process. Many of the positive effects of Chi Kung are directly related to this extra replenishment of oxygen and removal of waste products. Advanced Chi Kung practitioners can have an oxygen/carbon dioxide exchange rate ten times that of the average non-practitioner.

Chi Kung breathing, by its nature, affects the heart and circulatory system. Not only does it provide a cleaner product (fully cleaned and oxygenated blood) but also regulates the flow of that product both by the physical movement of the body tissues and the mental movement of Chi.

In Chinese Medicine it is believed that the Lungs control Chi and that Chi controls blood. Regulated breathing thus controls both Chi and Blood.

Various emotional conditions obviously affect the process of breathing. When you are calm, your breathing is "normal." Regulating the breath can help balance the emotions which aids in calming the mind.

Three major methods of breathing are used in Chi Kung: Normal, Natural and Reverse.

Normal breathing refers to regulating the quality and duration of the breath. Normal breathing is used in the Buddha Hands video.

In Natural breathing the lower abdomen expands with the inhale and contracts with the exhale. Some teachers recommend the expansion to include the whole area of the waist following the Belt Channel to stimulate both the Front-Lower Tan Tien and the Back-Ming Men. In Reverse Breathing the lower abdomen contracts with the inhale and expands with the exhale. This is considered the highest form of breathing by some teachers.

Both encourage the breath to be deep, slow, even, and soft. Deep refers to breathing to or from the area just below the navel (Lower Tan Tien). It is very important to concentrate your focus just below the navel and not in the whole lower abdomen.

According to my teacher, if the whole lower abdomen is used an imbalance will occur in the Urinary Bladder which can result in the development of a fat lower abdomen and high blood pressure.

Inhaling causes the Chi to rise and contract—exhaling causes the Chi to sink and expand. It is best to breath through the nose. This warms the air and stimulates nerve endings in the nose that benefit many organs, tissues, and functions of the body including heart rate, blood pressure, and the respiratory muscles.

Some specific Chi Kung exercises require breathing through the mouth. The danger of breathing through the mouth is that the mouth has a direct link to the stomach. Opening that link brings the possibility of losing digestive energy.

After a substantial period of deep regulated breathing there will be a gradual reduction in the amount of energy used in respiration which will further help the body relax.

Deep abdominal breathing massages the internal organs in the thorax and the abdomen and benefits the function of the cerebral cortex through the nerve reflexes.

2 | REGULATING BODY

R EGULATING THE BODY involves using posture to facilitate the flow of Chi within the body and/or receive and discharge Chi from outside the body more efficiently. Regulation of the body helps the mind to relax and relaxation of the mind helps the body to relax. During active relaxation, energy restoration in the body is promoted.

Particular body positions and/or movements cause specific manifestations of Chi flow in the body. This manifestation takes place both from the body position itself and the relative proximity of one part of the body to another.

When powerful energy centers (acupuncture points) pass other areas of the body they can induce Chi flow in those areas. This is especially true if there is a direct energetic connection between the two parts or if they have similar energetic qualities.

Rising postures cause the Chi to rise—lowering postures cause the Chi to sink—opening postures cause the Chi to disperse—closing postures cause the Chi to gather.

The holding of any posture causes some muscles to contract while other muscles relax. This causes various changes in the flow of Chi and Blood to various areas of the body which accounts for the efficacy of the posture.

3 | REGULATING MIND

R EGULATING THE MIND is the most important of the three regulations. In fact, the other regulations already employ regulation of the mind.

Substitute One Thought for a Thousand Thoughts

Disease and stress create imbalance in the excitement/inhibition responses of our nervous system. Calming the mind with a single thought can produce a deep inhibitory state (rest) for the cerebral cortex. This offers the nervous system an opportunity to regulate its function and thereby improve our health. Often the therapeutic results of Chi Kung practice can be related to this phenomenon.

Chi follows the mind, therefore the mind can lead Chi. Leading the Chi with the mind is perhaps the most powerful aspect of Chi Kung. Body position, movement and breath all affect the flow of Chi in the body, but the mind is the single most important factor in directing Chi. The mind is unlimited. Focusing the mind on Chi or an acupoint can effect body physiology. The cerebrum supplies bio-electric energy to the tissues of the body. When the mind focuses on one area the dermal electricity increases in that area and decreases in surrounding tissues.

Some systems of Chi Kung require the practitioner to use the mind to lead Chi along a specific channel. This method is used to reinforce the flow of Chi in specific areas. Other systems require the practitioner to focus the mind on a distal area and expect the Chi to follow the natural course to that area. Both methods work and each has its strong and weak points.

The strong point of leading the Chi is that it will strongly augment the flow if the practitioner truly knows the course of the channel. The weak point is, of course, that if the exact channel pathway is not known the flow of Chi may actually be retarded.

The strong point of using a distal point of focus is that the Chi can follow its natural pathway. The weak point is that the Chi may not flow as powerfully.

TECHNIQUES

TECHNIQUES in this context does not refer to specific movements or exercises but to considerations both inside and outside the exercises themselves.

SITE

CHOOSING A QUIET, pleasant and nurturing site will greatly enhance your practice. Some form of Chi Kung can be practiced almost anywhere and in later stages of development the practitioner will often practice throughout the routines of daily life.

The most important factor in location of the site is the availability of fresh air. Breath is one of the three regulations and air is an important source of energetic nutrition. One might say that you are what you breath.

Practicing in a forest, especially a pine forest, is ideal. Any area with lots of healthy greenery and low pollution is fine. Areas near oceans, lakes, or streams are also beneficial providing the atmosphere is not overly damp.

A modest knowledge of Feng Shui is invaluable in choosing a good practice area.

The ability to quiet your mind and ask yourself how you feel in a certain spot is important. Your body/mind/spirit will know whether a place "feels" right or not. For those who must practice indoors, seek a well ventilated room that you feel comfortable in and keep the room clean.

Grave sites are not auspicious places to practice, nor are areas with withered vegetation. Avoid extremes of heat, cold, wind, and damp. Chi Kung should not be practiced during heavy storms especially with thunder and lightning.

DIRECTION

THERE ARE MANY THEORIES regarding the direction to face while practicing Chi Kung. As with site selection, one totally valid method is to quietly "feel" each direction and face the one in which you are most comfortable. You should feel outwardly stable and inwardly responsive as you quiet your mind and face the proper direction.

My teacher recommends facing the sun in the daytime and the moon at night.

Similar Chi's support and seek each other. South and East are considered Yang directions and North and West are considered Yin.

One school of thought suggests facing South or East to strengthen Yang and North or West to strengthen Yin. East relates to the wood element which represents growth. Since Chi Kung practitioners are attempting to grow their Chi, East is a popular direction to face especially in the morning as the sun (Yang) is rising.

Another school of thought looks at the front of the body as Yin and the back as Yang. Yin has sedating and downward qualities while Yang has tonifying and upward qualities. This school would face South and East to nourish Yin and face North and West to nourish Yang.

The directions are also associated with organs. East relates to the Liver—North to the Kidneys—South to the Heart—and West to the Lungs.

If one had weak Kidneys and excess Fire in the Heart which is common in chronic disease, he could face South.

The front of the body being Yin and facing South, the direction of the Heart which represents fire, would draw the Heart fire down. The back being Yang and facing North, the direction of the Kidneys, would bring Kidney energy up.

Using this theory a person with an excess Liver and deficient Lungs would face East. East is the direction of the Liver and the front of the body is Yin. The Liver excess would be brought down and the Lung energy would be brought up as the back of the body would face West.

With all these theories it may be difficult for the novice—or even an expert—to really know intellectually which direction is best. This brings us back to the "feeling" method, which is simple and effective, or simply following the sun or moon.

One last point concerning direction is that if an exercise moves to both left and right sides from the center and one begins to the right side the exercise is generally more tonifying while if one begins to the left side the exercise is generally more sedative in nature.

MOVEMENT

UPWARD MOVEMENTS make the Chi rise—downward movements make the Chi sink—opening movements spread Chi from the interior to the exterior—closing movements concentrate Chi from the extremities to the interior. These are the ways Chi is influenced by movement.

An excess of spreading will cause the Chi to dissipate and an excess of closing movements will cause the Chi to stagnate. Likewise, an excess of either upward or downward movements will cause imbalances in the respected direction of Chi flow.

Inhaling makes the Chi rise and concentrate while exhaling makes the Chi sink and spread to the extremities.

Chi Kung exercises use a combination of breath co-ordination and physical movement to regulate Chi flow in the desired manner, but the most important regulation is the mind.

In exercises requiring very powerful Chi flows, the mind, breath, and body movements may all co-ordinate to produce Chi flow in one direction. Often, in order to moderate Chi flow one of the three regulations may actually restrain the flow to create a better balance of Yin and Yang. For the same reason (balance) exercises are often performed on both the left and right sides.

When one body part, particularly if a potent acupuncture point is involved, moves past another body part or comes in close proximity to another part, the flow of Chi will be affected. The closer the distance and the closer the energetic connection between the two parts the greater the effect.

For instance raising your hand from foot to chest will cause Chi to rise in your body and lowering your hand from chest to foot will cause the Chi to sink. If your hand is closer to your body while rising than it is when descending the overall result of the two movements will be a rise in Chi (assuming your regulated mind wills the rise). Often Chi Kung exercises contain more than one type of movement. The different types of movement restrain and promote each other, each being the prerequisite for the other. In these exercises breath, body movement and mind all modulate and harmonize each other to produce the desired effect. Systems of Chi Kung often have a variety of combinations.

Another type of movement that affects Chi in Chi Kung exercises involves the movement of soft-connective tissue. When muscles and tendons flex and contract over an acupuncture point, they activate the functions of that point. Depending on how many flexion/ contraction cycles are performed the point will be either tonified, sedated or harmonized.

The Eighteen Buddha Hands Chi Kung requires eight repetitions of each movement which generally allows the function of the points to express themselves according to the body's needs.

Regarding the movements of air while breathing, long exhaling brings Chi down and reduces blood pressure by expanding blood vessels in the extremities while long inhaling brings Chi up and constricts blood vessels in the extremities.

People with excess conditions in the top and deficiency below should exhale longer than inhaling and of course those with upper deficiencies should inhale longer than exhaling.

Remember these are all general rules:

The Mind Is The Most Important Regulator!

In most cases the final step in any Chi Kung exercise should be to guide the Chi back to the Lower Tan Tien.

TIME

SPRING AND SUMMER ARE YANG SEASONS while Fall and Winter are considered Yin. It is easier to nourish Yang Chi in the Spring and Summer and to nourish Yin Chi in the Fall and Winter.

Morning is considered Yang and afternoon is considered Yin. It is easier to nourish Yang in the morning and Yin in the afternoon. Generally in Chi Kung the morning is the best time to train because the Chi by nature is aroused and growing at that time.

Most systems of Chi Kung are balanced in such a way that training any time is appropriate.

Training Any Time Is Better Than No Time!

Environmentally the Chi is changing its yin/yang nature at sunrise, midday, sunset, and midnight. These are good times to train Chi Kung as the body can take advantage of the environmental changes to help make internal changes.

A "crest" of Chi moves through the Twelve Primary Meridians in each twenty-four hour period spending two hours in each meridian system. If a practitioner has a disharmony in one of the meridian systems it is beneficial (if not convenient) to practice Chi Kung during the time of that system.

THE TIMES ARE:
Lung: 3—5 am | Large Intestine: 5—7 am | Stomach: 7—9 am
Spleen: 9—11 am | Heart: 11 am—1 pm | Small Intestine: 1—3 pm
Urinary Bladder: 3—5 pm | Kidney: 5—7 pm
Pericardium: 7—9 pm | Triple Burner: 9—11 pm
Gall Bladder: 11 pm—1 am | Liver: 1—3 am

ABSORBING ENERGY FROM NATURE

THERE ARE SEVERAL important points on the human body where the internal energy of man can directly connect with the energy of the environment. These points are often used in Chi Kung practice to absorb supplemental energy from nature and to release excess or toxic energy from the body. These points will be discussed in detail in a later section.

COLOR

COLOR THERAPY can be used with Chi Kung practice. If the practitioner has a disharmony with one of his organ systems the color associated with that system can be utilized during daily practice. Any material of the appropriate color can be hung in view of the practitioner during practice. Viewing natural objects of the appropriate color is even better. Color therapy can be applied to the various Five Element strategies of Chinese Medicine but should not be attempted without the consultation of a knowledgeable Doctor.

- RED is the color corresponding to the Heart, Small Intestine, Pericardium, and Triple Heater

- YELLOW is the color corresponding to the Spleen and Stomach

- WHITE is the color corresponding to the Lungs and Large Intestine

- BLACK is the color corresponding to the Kidneys and Urinary Bladder

- GREEN is the color corresponding to the Liver and Gall Bladder.

CHAPTER 3

Taoist Chi Kung

THE GENERAL FORMULA for Taoist Spiritual/Energetic practices is: (A) to refine and transform Jing to Chi (B) to refine and transform Chi to Shen (C) to return Shen to Nothingness (D) to extinguish nothingness. This is a linear description of processes that are concurrently operating in every human being all the time. Unfortunately these processes are compromised at birth by the desires and expectations of our minds and the assaults of the external world. Taoist Chi Kung practices restore the natural flow of these processes and reverse accumulated damage both from the external environment and the mind. The end result of this training is to produce a Natural Man—one through which the unlimited potential of the universe manifests without contrivance.

Jing, Chi, and Shen are considered the three treasures of man and each is associated with one of the three main energy centers of the body. Jing is associated with the Lower Tan Tien—just below the navel, Chi is associated with the Middle Tan Tien—middle of the chest, and Shen is associated with the Upper Tan Tien—mid-eyebrow.

JING

THE CHINESE CHARACTER representing Jing is composed of two parts. The part on the left represents a grain of rice or other cereal that is bursting. The part on the right represents the color of life—usually thought of as a rich vibrant green. Together these parts represent materials that can sustain, rebuild and support life. Jing is a subtle element (essence) that can be absorbed from another source through which one can replenish the material body at its most refined level.

Usually we gather these essences through the digestive process, but advanced Chi Kung practitioners can absorb essence through direct communication with outside sources. Essences are the components of life on a much subtler level than the molecules of the food we eat. They are the substrate that forms the model of our physical being, inseparable from the organizational structure of our life. Every part of our development from the embryo through our adult forms is organized by Jing.

Our initial organization comes from Before Heaven Jing—provided by our parents. Later organization comes from After Heaven Jing which results from our personal transformation and assimilation of essences from the outside.

Although Jing, Chi, and Shen are spoken of separately, in a human being each is intimately and inseparably connected with the others. Essences have no purpose without being transformed—transformation being a function of Chi. Chi on the other hand is sustained, held, and birthed from Essence. The foundations of Chi and Jing are oriented by Shen, which directs all circulations and transformations.

Jing is especially linked to the Kidneys and reproductive energy. Reproduction is the passing on of a model of being (one model from each parent joining) and Jing represents the purest representation of the individual model. Through the transformational activity of Chi, Jing is responsible for building and rebuilding all the physical structures of the body. Jing has no form itself, but rather is the condition for form to materialize.

CHI

THE CHINESE CHARACTER for Chi contains the same bursting grain as the character for Jing, but to that part is added the symbol for exhalation indicating movement. The term Chi is used to describe various energies and those energies have a definite quality ascribed to them. For instance the Chi of the Lungs, or the Chi of a tree, or the Chi of Heaven, etc.

Inside the human body, Chi is both a carrier and a message. It transfers both energy and information. Emitted Chi from Chi Kung Masters has been proven to contain infrared radiation, particle streams, static electricity, etc.

The seven basic functions of Chi in the body are:

1. **Chi** *is transformative—it activates all the organic functions of the body*

2. **Chi** *moves blood and fluids throughout the body*

3. **Chi** *is the basic source of warmth for the body*

4. **Chi** *defends the body from exterior factors*

5. **Chi** *holds the various fluids and tissues in place in the body*

6. **Chi** *of the Kidney is in charge of reproduction*

7. **Chi** *controls the overall coordinated functioning of the body*

The five main classifications of Chi in the body are:

1. **Source Chi** is the chi we inherit from our parents. It is our basic constitutional energy. Stored in our Kidneys, Source Chi stimulates all of our functions and when it is exhausted, we die.

2. **Ancestral Chi** is composed of the air we breath and the essences of the food and water we consume. Stored in the chest, it is responsible for the rhythms and power of respiration and the flow of blood in the Heart.

3. **Central Chi** is our basic digestive energy. All the organs of the body depend on adequate Central Chi to function properly.

4. **Constructive Chi** is obtained through the digestive process. It moves with the blood and nourishes our entire body.

5. **Defensive Chi** moves outside the vessels, nourishing the subcutaneous tissues, controlling the opening and closing of pores, warming the skin and muscles and defending the body from external factors.

In terms of the Taoist Chi Kung formula, it is the transformative functions of Chi that resonate with the references to "Chi." In this case we are not talking about the usual transformations that are part and parcel of normal life functions. We are talking about transformations at a deeper level in the body/mind/Spirit complex.

After balancing and strengthening the normal life processes through work at the Jing Level, activating potential energies beyond the normal scope of everyday living is the next step in the alchemical transformation process.

SHEN

SHEN, which is translated as Spirit, is nourished by both Jing and Chi. It is the force of our consciousness and thought processes. Shen is the guidance system for the whole body and is closely associated with both the Heart and the brain. It controls our physical energies and thought processes both conscious and subconscious.

Although Shen controls both Jing and Chi, injury to either will adversely affect Shen.

The processes of refining Jing, Chi and Shen constitute the pathway to self-realization—Spiritual evolution.

HUA SHAN TAOIST CHI KUNG

IN OUR SYSTEM, the Taoist formula for Spiritual evolution mentioned above is simply presented as three groups of thirty six exercises each. The first group helps to prevent and eliminate sickness—refining and transforming Jing. The second group is said to return one's youthfulness from old age—refining and transforming Chi. The third group will help tranquilize the mind and harmonize the will, thus achieving longevity with a strong, healthy body and clear, tranquil mind—leading to the return of Shen to nothingness. The fourth stage, as indicated above, is related more to receiving grace than to actively pursuing it. In other words, direct experience of the Divine can not be contrived. Rather the first three stages set the stage for that oneness to spontaneously manifest.

To understand the pathways of Hua Shan Taoist Chi Kung, we must look at the overall energetic potentials—both manifest and unmanifest of the human being.

In theory, there are four basic degrees of human realization/potential.

The first degree is represented by the Divine Spirit. It is the state of singularity beyond Yin and Yang. Reaching this state is the highest aim of Spiritual Enlightenment.

The second degree is represented by the harmonious interaction of Yin and Yang. Both principles are present but have not yet differentiated. This is the level of the Source/Ming Men—origin of the Pericardium/Triple Burner duality.

The third degree is where Yin and Yang differentiate to manifest Water and Fire—their basic representatives in Man.

The fourth degree embodies the results from the activities and interactions of Water and Fire. These include the Five Elemental (Phase) Energies, the Eight Extra-Ordinary Vessels, the Twelve Regular Meridians, and all the structures, rhythms and functions of the body.

The pathway of development in Hua Shan Chi Kung leads the practitioner from the fourth degree upwards to ultimately unite with the Divine.

LEVEL 1 | **Essence**—exercises work at the level of the fourth degree, supporting proper functioning of all the energies and functions at that level.

LEVEL 2 | **Chi**—exercises work at the level of the third degree, supporting the transforming interactions of Water and Fire that provide more refined energies to approach higher consciousness.

LEVEL 3 | **Shen**—exercises address the co-penetration of the refined energies from Level 2 with the embodied Spirit of the individual to open the doorway for reception of Divine Grace.

Ancient pathways to Spiritual development from many cultures require a lot of time, effort and a complete system with which to work. It is always emphasized that each stage of the way must be completed before a more advanced stage should be undertaken, and that there is a specifically prescribed method and timing for the process. It is my belief that these 108 exercises are an exact outline of the what, how, and when of a complete system that has been orally passed down for thousands of years. Although other systems may approach these stages differently, I believe any complete system should contain some version of the areas covered by these exercises to develop safely and effectively.

Whereas the energetic history of this system is long, the intellectual history is scanty. My Sifu, Chan Chiu Lim, learned from his teacher on a mountain in China. His teacher had no name. "He was natural, like a rock or a tree" was the reply to my question regarding that name. The only other information passed down to me on the system is that Lao Tsu may have studied it. When he left China, my Sifu truly believed that his teacher was 180 years old. ☯

CHAPTER 4

Exercises for Level One: Refining and Transforming Jing

WARNING!
The information provided for these exercises is for educational
purposes only. No attempt should be made to learn or practice
these exercises without the personal attention of a qualified
chi kung instructor. The author, publisher, and distributors
of this work can accept no responsibility for any use
or misuse of this information by the reader.

THE BEGINNING STAGES of training Hua Shan Taoist Chi Kung involve practicing the exercises a very specific number of times each day. When my teacher learned this stage, the exercises were taught one per month. Now they are generally taught one per week, so it is extremely important to practice according to the correct schedule in order to build a strong foundation for later work.

The numbering system is as follows: when the practitioner has one exercise he does it thirty six times, three times a day. When he has two exercises he does them eighteen times each, three times a day. Each succeeding number of exercises is done the highest multiple of times that does not exceed thirty six. For instance when the practitioner has seven exercises he does them five times each three times a day. After eighteen exercises they are each done once, three times a day.

The best results are obtained through regular daily training. There is no "getting it right." The effects of the exercises become more profound as they accumulate through regular practice. Training over many years continues to refine the techniques and in turn the techniques eventually refine the practitioner. The effects of the exercises are not necessarily limited to the Level in which they are placed. As the practitioner advances, Level One exercises may elicit Level Two or Level Three responses. Ultimately, the three levels are one so any exercise can effect any level. The exercises are presented in the Three Levels to "order the firing process" which enables a safe and complete developmental process.

THE CHI IS UNLIMITED!

1.1 | BASIC

In some ways, the Basic is the most important exercise in the system

IT IS DESIGNED to balance all the energy in the body and eliminate toxins of all kinds. With that in mind, it automatically follows every other exercise, so is performed more than any other. Proficiency in the Basic is absolutely necessary for the safe development of the practitioner.

The initial inhale and hand movements gather to the chest any toxins released in the body by other exercises. The head is held back to prevent toxin from the lower body rising past the chest. The next hand movement collects toxin from the head. Then everything is expelled by bending forward and exhaling. The bending and exhaling functions both to help release toxin and to rebalance—center—the body's energy. In later stages of training the Basic is modified somewhat to focus more on moving toxin through the body to the ground and cleaning the bones.

Because it centers the energy, the Basic supports the Spleen—related to the Earth (center)—element. The bending activates the Kidney, storehouse of the fundamental constitutional energy.

It is interesting to note that almost all the inhalations and exhalations in the system modulate the air with the nose—the tip of the nose is slightly contracted. Ancient Taoists believed that the first energy to form in the body was the Ming Men and the first cells were those of the nose. The tip of the nose was thought to be directly related to the Ming Men. In the present day practice of acupuncture, the tip of the nose can be used to treat the spine and acute lumbar sprain (Ming Men area). It is also used to restore consciousness. The point is able to redirect the route of elimination of liver toxins to the lungs thus making exhalations more effective as cleansing strategies.

STRATEGY NOTE | *The main functions of the Yin organs are to manufacture and store essential substances such as vital essence, vital energy and body fluids. They take the products of digestion and refine them to match the particular quality of the individual person, thus "storing" is much more than simply holding essence. It is a dynamic function impossible to divorce from the life process. The five elements, in relation to the Yin organs, indicate that there are five ways to acquire and categorize essences. Representing your deeper self, the Yin organs perform this function. Appropriately, Taoist Chi Kung begins with invigorating and harmonizing the five Yin organs*

1.2 | MONKEY
Cleans and Harmonizes the Liver

SINCE THE LIVER corresponds to the energy of Spring—the impetus for the expansion of life—it is an appropriate beginning exercise. The Liver is associated with the Wood Element and the Eastern direction.

The Liver stores blood. When we are not active, the Liver stores a certain amount of blood and when the blood is needed it is released. Both the Liver and Heart are instrumental in supplying blood to the tissues and organs. Naturally the Liver has a strong influence on menstruation. The Liver's influence on the overall energetic state of the body is directly reflected in its ability to regulate the quantity and distribution of the blood. This function of storing blood brings the Liver into close association with the

Chong Mai—Sea of Blood—Central Channel. It is interesting to note that the Liver Channel has an internal branch that reaches the top of the head (GV 20) and the Central Channel—main pathway for Spiritual Development—directly accesses the same point.

The Liver is in charge of the free-flow of Chi throughout the body. It is especially prevalent in the spreading and elevation of Chi and the removal of obstacles. This function affects the activities of the Spleen/Stomach in the process of digestion and absorption, the Gall Bladder in its function of bile storage and secretion into the Small Intestine, and the emotional activities of the body. Anger is the emotion associated with the Liver but any emotion that is out of balance will disrupt the smooth flow of Chi in the body and ultimately affect the Liver.

The Liver controls the tendons. Yin organs store essences, and the essences associated directly with the Liver are those relating to the tendons and connective tissues of the body. Although strength is based in the Kidneys, the manifestation of strength is related to the Liver. It functions at the beginning of all movements.

Manifesting in the nails, the Liver also has a close relationship with the eyes due to direct channel connections.

The practitioner begins by raising his hands from the sides to the level of the head—thus activating the upward flow of energy in the body. The arms are then brought together in front of the body with the forearms touching from fist to elbow. This gathers the rising energy and condenses it in the area of the liver. At the same time the legs bend lightly to root and support the energy from beneath, the lower spine is gently tucked in to open the lower spine, the upper back is slightly rounded to facilitate energy flow in the mid—spine, and the chin is tucked to open the upper spine.

This tucking of the chin and lower spine and rounding of the back is a recurrent theme throughout this system and Chi Kung in general. The actions result in minimizing the inward curvatures of the neck and low back thus "bowing" the spine. The "bow" elongates the spine, thus opening the intervertebral spaces and increasing the ability of the subtle channels in the area to conduct energy. This position is the Chi Kung version of the three Bandhas of Yoga.

The three Bandhas are positions in which muscles are controlled in such a way as to produce a psychomuscular energy lock which directs the flow of energy in the body and locks energy in specific places. The Chi Kung bowed spine position is not as extreme as the bandha positions and is concerned with facilitating flow of energy rather than locking it. Pranayama—yogic breath control—is said to be incomplete without the practice of the three bandhas either together or in various combinations.

Jalandhara Bandha, Uddiyana Bandha and Moola Bandha are the names of these positions. Proper practice of the three bandhas awakens the dormant Kundalini (spiritual energy, capacity, and consciousness) and allows it to enter the Sushumna (main channel in the center of the spinal cord). In time the breath stills, the senses become purified and enlightenment takes place.

Jalandhara bandha, or the "throat-lock," requires the chin to rest forward on the sternum. It is said to directly influence the functioning of the pituitary, pineal, thyroid, parathyroid, and thymus glands.

Uddiyana bandha, or the "abdominal retraction lock," requires the stomach and abdomen to be drawn inwards toward the spine. It is said to directly influence the adrenals and pancreas.

Moola Bandha requires the contraction of the perineal body in the male and the cervix in the female. It is said to directly influence the gonads and perineal body/cervix—which are believed to be vestigial endocrine glands.

The Taoist Traditions have three "gates" which are considered places along the spine that energy flows are restricted. This bowed spine position facilitates the opening of these three gates. Most authorities place two of the gates at the coccyx area and where the spine meets the head. Authorities differ on the location of the middle gate, placing it in the lower back (GV 4), mid back (GV 9) or upper back (GV 14).

Returning to the Monkey, when the correct position is achieved a smooth clear hissing sound is made through the mouth. The hissing sound cools, expels toxin from and moves energy through the liver.

The correct posture is very important to support the cleansing action of the Monkey. Each organ is said to be generated from a "mother" organ and in turn generates a "son" organ. The Liver is generated by the Kidneys, and generates the Heart. The specific energetic quality of the Kidneys that gives rise to the Liver is the marrow. The greatest repositories of marrow in the body are the brain (marrow defined as that which is encased in bone) and spinal cord. As we have seen, the "bowed" position of the spine facilitates energy flow in the whole spinal column.

The position of the hands places bilateral acupoints SI 3 together, thus stimulating them. This acupoint controls the Governing Vessel which runs up the midline of the back and has an enormous impact on the spine.

1.3 | THE DRAGON
Cleans and Harmonizes the Heart

The Heart is associated with the energy of Summer, the Fire Element and the Southern direction.

The Heart controls the blood and the blood vessels. It is also said to "house the mind" and is the organ most associated with consciousness, memory, thinking, and sleep. The Heart opens to the tongue, governs sweating, and its energy manifests in the complexion.

The Heart is regarded as the Emperor, regulating the activities of the whole body through the influences of the Divine Spirits which reside therein. In some ancient Chi Kung writings, it is stated that if one can regulate the Heart no other exercise is needed to maintain good health.

The Dragon begins with the practitioner raising his open hands from the sides to the level of the head while inhaling—bringing energy up in the body. Since the Heart belongs to the Fire Element and Fire energy naturally rises and spreads, this movement activates Heart energy.

Next the practitioner inhales again while squatting low and bringing closed hands down to the thighs. This action gathers the Fire energy and brings it down in the body to meet the Water energy residing in the lower abdomen. Fire and Water balance and support each other. Their meeting both keeps the body harmonized and in more advanced levels of practice (Level Two) initiates Spiritual transformations.

From this position, the practitioner springs up raising the hands overhead and exhaling the specific sound for cleansing the Heart. The Liver is said to generate the Heart, and the specific energetic quality of the Liver that accomplishes this is the Liver's muscle—animating energy. This movement uses that animating force to nourish the Heart while simultaneously cleansing the Heart with sound.

The exercise is completed with two more repetitions of the inhale/squat—exhale/upward thrust motion.

1.4 | TIGER

Cleans and Harmonizes the Lungs

The Lungs are associated with the Element Metal and the Western direction.

The main functions of the Lungs are to dominate Chi and control respiration. Through its dispersing and descending actions, the Lungs take in clean air and remove wastes, affecting the Chi of the whole body. They also regulate the water passages of the body, turning part of the body fluid to sweat and dispersing it to the skin and sending part of the body fluids down to the Kidney for excretion. The dispersing action also nourishes the skin and regulates the pores.

The Lungs are also said to control physical energy. This is accomplished through their increasing or decreasing the rate and depth of respiration, and through their transformation process. In this transformation process, the essences of food (from the Spleen) rises to the Lungs to be combined with "Heavenly Energy" inhaled by the Lungs. This mixture is then transformed to create Chen Chi—energy required by the body for normal functions.

The entire Tiger exercise is done with "Tiger Claw Hands." In this hand position, the four fingers are bent so the tips are touching the distal edge of the palm. The thumb is bent and spread to the side. The palm is spread resulting in an opening of the energy passages in the chest. This hand position is used in several exercises in the system, always to increase energy flow to the chest—Lungs/Heart.

The exercise begins with the practitioner raising his hands as he inhales—bringing energy up in the body. He then bends his legs and brings his hands to the sides of the chest—gathering the energy in and expanding the chest. Next the hands are thrust out at shoulder level and the legs straighten while the practitioner exhales the Tiger sound. This motion is done with tension in the arms and legs. As in all exercises, a Basic follows.

The natural tendency of Lung energy is to contract and press down. To aid in the cleansing action of the sound associated with the Lung, the physical action of the Tiger activates the Son of the Lung—Kidney by using muscle tension to drive the Chi into the bones, which relate to and are controlled by the Kidneys.

1.5 | HAWK

Cleans and Strengthens the Kidneys

THE KIDNEYS are associated with the Water element and the Northern direction.

The Kidneys store Essence and dominate reproduction, growth and development. They produce marrow, dominate the bones, fill the brain (brain=Sea of Marrow) and assist in blood production. Kidneys also control water and the reception of Chi.

In Chinese Medicine the Lungs inhale air, but the Kidneys "root" that air in the body. The Kidneys are the storehouse of energy for the body, and in some traditions are never directly cleaned. It is considered dangerous to take anything out of the Kidneys directly as this might cause a loss of "good" energy along with the "bad." The Hawk does not utilize sound to clean the Kidneys, but does stimulate the son—Liver—to flush out toxins. This is especially important in the Jing Level. In the Chi Level an exercise called the Bear does use sound to clean the Kidneys, but by this stage of training the body will naturally differentiate the "good" from the "bad."

The exercise begins with the practitioner bent 90° at the waist with arms hanging down and hands in fists. He stands up inhaling while spreading the arms to the sides at shoulder level—bringing energy up in the body and expanding the chest—POOH.

Next the practitioner turns from side to side six times while alternately swinging the arms overhead and inhaling on each turn. This involves six inhales without any exhales—very difficult for the beginning practitioner. The repeated inhaling exercises the Kidneys' ability to root air in the body. The low spread out stance utilized while turning aids the Kidneys in rooting and the vigorous upward swinging arm motions stimulate the natural rising energy of the Liver while providing further expansiveness for the chest.

Although this exercise seems impossible to beginners, steady practice of the system teaches the body to utilize air in unusual ways, thus allowing for multiple inhales.

1.6 | ENERGY TO THE FOUR LIMBS
Supports and Harmonizes the Spleen

THE SPLEEN is associated with the Earth element and the Central position.

The Spleen governs transportation and transformation. Transformation refers to the digestion of food and absorption of essential nutrients and fluids. Transportation refers to transmitting "pure essences" to the Heart and Lungs where they combine with inhaled air to form Chi for use by the body. The transforming and transporting functions of the Spleen allow adequate nourishment for the muscles, so the Spleen is said to dominate the muscles and control the energy in the four limbs.

The Spleen is also said to produce blood and keep the blood in the vessels.

This exercise is also done entirely with Tiger Claw Hands. Although Energy to the four Limbs is not physically complicated, it utilizes energies of all the Elements to support and harmonize the center—Spleen. The Tiger Claw Hands are used to bring Heart (the Mother) and Lung (the Son) energies into the exercise.

The exercise begins with the practitioner's right leg stretched out and the left leg bent and holding most of the bodyweight. The left hand is on the left side of the waist and the right hand hangs at the right side.

The right hand is raised up about 135° while inhaling and then dropped to 90° (parallel to the ground at chest level) while holding the breath—activating the Heart (upward—expanding) and Lung (downward—contracting) energies. The right hand is then brought across the chest to the left shoulder—activating the Lung through acupoints LU 1 and LU 2 and both the Lung and Liver by physically contracting the chest and activating the "spreading" quality of the Wood—Liver energy. Returning the right hand to the previous position enhances the effect.

The hand is then dropped to the thigh—activating the most downward moving energy in the body—Kidney. From this position, the practitioner lunges to the right and extends his arm out at shoulder level, then pulls the right hand back to his waist while drawing his right leg back towards the left leg so there is no weight on the right leg. Again the practitioner lunges to the right, this time with great vigor while exhaling and extending the right arm out at shoulder level. These last body motions encourage Blood and Chi circulation in the limbs by the weight shifting and vigorous thrusting movements. The waist turning involved also stimulates the Kidneys.

The Earth—Spleen—is said to appear through the crossing of the vertical movements of Water—Kidneys—to Fire—Heart—and the horizontal movements of Wood—Liver to Metal—Lungs. Energy to the Four Limbs activates all these energetic movements in the body and pumps the muscles through vigorous movements and weight sifts to emphasize the Spleen.

STRATEGY NOTE | *The Pericardium and Triple Burner are different from the other organ/functions. They have a "name but no form." They are precursors to all the element, organ, and meridian relationships. The Triple Burner is said to be the Yang Chi of the father and the Pericardium is said to be the Yin Chi of the mother. The mechanisms of these two link the entire body to Source Chi and the influence of the Spirits.*

1.7 | HORSE RIDING 1
Strengthens and Harmonizes the Pericardium

THE PERICARDIUM is a fatty membrane that surrounds the Heart. Energetically it functions as a protector of the Heart. The Pericardium belongs to the Fire Element and is related to the South.

The exercise begins with the practitioner standing with his feet at shoulder width and hands at the sides. He raises his hands to the level of the head, thus bringing the energy in the body upwards. Next the practitioner drops his fists to the sides of his chest while bending the knees. The original raising of the arms stimulated the Fire energy in the body. The positioning of the fists at the chest collects that Fire energy in the Pericardium and the bending of the knees activates Water energy which balances the Fire. (Fire energy rises and expands while Water energy sinks and contracts).

At this time the sound POOH is made by expelling air through the mouth. This sound is often used in Taoist Chi Kung to protect the Heart. Many exercises in this system use both external muscular tension and internal air pressure to accomplish their goals. It is necessary to use the POOH sound to ensure Chi does not congest in the Heart/chest.

Next the hands are opened and the arms are fully extended outwards at shoulder level with tension while inhaling. This inhale and extension serves to "fill up" the Pericardium channel (runs from chest to the tip of the middle finger) while the tension collects Chi in the arms and leads the Chi to the bones, activating Kidney—Water Chi to balance the Fire. The hands return to fists and are drawn back to the chest with tension while holding the breath. This packs the Chi from the channel into the Pericardium itself.

The practitioner then bends forward at 90°, opens his fists and extends his arms backward parallel to the ground with tension while inhaling. Again the tension activates Water Chi and the inhale and extension fills the Pericardium channel.

The hands are returned to fists and pulled back to the chest while holding the breath. The Pericardium is further packed with Chi.

From the chest the fists are pushed towards the floor in a "Half Basic" while exhaling. This is followed by a normal Basic.

This exercise is very powerful, fully activating the Fire Chi of the Pericardium and using both the bending of the back and tension to activate Kidney/Water Chi for balance and support.

1.8 | HORSE RIDING 2
Strengthens and Harmonizes the Triple Burner

THE TRIPLE BURNER is a generalization of the functions of the organs in three areas of the body. The Upper Burner represents the chest and functions of the Heart and Lungs in transporting Blood and Chi. The Middle Burner represents the epigastrium and the functions of the Spleen/Stomach in digestion and absorption. The Lower Burner represents the hypogastrium and functions of the Kidney/Urinary Bladder and Large Intestine in controlling water metabolism and the excretion of waste products. The Triple Burner belongs to the Fire Element and is related to the South.

Beyond the obvious functional responsibilities outlined above, the Triple Burner plays a germain role in all activities of the body. Ming Men is the Original energy of life and Yin (Water) and Yang (Fire) are the first differentiation of that energy in the living being. The Triple Burner is the vehicle through which the interactions of that first differentiation build and support life. It links whatever follows to the Source and extends the power of the Source throughout the body. The Triple Burner transports Jing, Chi and Shen throughout the body.

The exercise begins with the practitioner standing with his feet at shoulder width and hands at the sides. He raises his hands to the level of the head, thus bringing the energy in the body upwards. Next the practitioner drops his fists to the sides of his chest while bending the knees. The original raising of the arms stimulated the Fire energy in the body. The positioning of the fists at the chest collects that Fire energy in the chest and the bending of the knees activates Water energy which balances the Fire. (Fire energy rises and expands while Water energy sinks and contracts).

At this time the sound POOH is made by expelling air through the mouth.

The fists are then opened and the hands pushed overhead with tension while inhaling. This motion fills the upper body with Fire Chi while the tension both collects Chi and activates Water/Kidney Chi from the bones to balance the Fire. The hands are again formed into fists and returned to the front of the chest without breathing and with tension—collecting the Fire Chi in the chest.

The practitioner then bends forward at 90°. The fists open and the hands are extended downwards and to the sides with tension while inhaling. The combination of the downward arm motion, the bending of the waist, and the second inhale serves to activate the Kidneys and bring the Fire Chi to the Water Chi.

The outstretched hands are turned to fists and returned to the chest with tension but no breathing. This harmonizes Fire and Water in the Triple Burner.

Finally the practitioner does a Half Basic and a Basic to complete the exercise.

1.9 | CENTERING THE ENERGY
Activates the Lower Tan Tien—Ming Men

THE LOWER TAN TIEN is located just below the navel. Authorities differ on its exact location and in fact the location can vary in different individuals. The perception of the location of the Lower Tan Tien can change for each individual at various stages of training. Complete Chi Kung systems will provide the tools for the student's relationship with the Lower Tan Tien to become closer and more exact as his practice matures.

The Lower Tan Tien is the foundation of the body. It not only stores the Original Chi (derived from parents at conception), but also acts as a storehouse where Chi from all sources is collected, blended and transformed.

Ming Men is the first and most important energy center in the body. First because it is formed at the moment of conception, even before the fetus is formed, and most important because it is the center of energetic transformations.

Bilateral Ming Men, located in the Kidneys, has seven energy channels connecting its two sides called the "Moving Chi between the Kidneys." This is where Heaven and Earth meet in Man and interact to produce life. Prenatal Chi, Postnatal Chi, and cosmic energy interface and transform in Ming Men to support life. It is the origin of the Governing Vessel, the Conception Vessel, Chong Mai, and the Triple Burner.

Ming Men is often considered the back of the Lower Tan Tien. In fact, the Lower Tan Tien, Moving Chi between the Kidneys and Ming Men are so intimately connected that they can be considered one.

The exercise begins with the practitioner standing with feet wide apart and waist bent forward so the body is parallel to the ground. The hands are held touching the waist with the middle fingers touching at the navel.

The practitioner straightens the waist while inhaling—filling the chest with air/energy. He then bends forward again and turns to the left while straightening the right leg and pressing the bent left knee over the left foot. At this point he exhales through the nose—gathering the energy from the chest to the Lower Tan Tien.

Now, keeping bent parallel to the ground, the practitioner turns to the right side straightening the left leg and pressing the bent right knee over the right foot. He then straightens the waist while inhaling—filling the chest with air/energy and bends forward to the parallel position. At this point he exhales through the nose—gathering the energy from the chest to the Lower Tan Tien.

This side to side process is repeated until three repetitions have been completed on each side. After the third exhale on the right side, the practitioner straightens up inhaling and after turning to the front performs a Half Basic followed by a Basic.

Turning from side to side utilizes the back muscles to stimulate the two side channels of Ming Men. The legs bring energy up from the earth to the Lower Tan Tien during the inhale phase of the exercise, where it is collected during the exhale. The bending up and down stimulates both the Lower Tan Tien and the Ming Men. This position also activates the Conception Vessel, Governing Vessel and Chong Mai. These vessels will be explained in more detail as we progress.

STRATEGY NOTE | *After learning the Basic, which is the protective ending for every other exercise, the practitioner has activated and balanced the five Yin organs. These organs constitute the deep layers of the body that deal with assimilation and matriculation of Essences. Next the Pericardium was activated to bring the commands from the spirits of the Heart more clearly into the overall system. Then the Triple Burner was addressed to link the energy from the Source to the rest of the body.*

Centering the Energy is the link between the initial Yin energy exercises and the upcoming Yang exercises. The Conception Vessel is said to control all the Yin of the body and the Governing Vessel controls the Yang. They both emanate from the Center and are activated by Centering the Energy. The system has begun by activating and harmonizing the deep Yin energies, clearing the energy and control channels and bringing attention to the Center. Now from the Center the more superficial Yang energies will be activated.

1.10 | TURTLE
Governing Vessel/Ming Men

THE GOVERNING VESSEL controls all the Yang of the body and is usually viewed as the channel that ascends through the spine to the brain (Sea of Marrow). A closer study of the vessel reveals that it actually has three branches. The first originates in the lower abdomen, descends to the perineum and genitals,

ascends the interior of the spinal column and enters the Kidneys.
The second branch originates in the lower abdomen, descends
to the external genitalia, ascends to the umbilicus, Heart, and
throat, winds around the mouth and terminates below the middle of the eyes. The final branch emerges at the inner canthus,
bilaterally follows the Urinary Bladder channel up the forehead
to the vertex where the two channels enter the brain. This branch
emerges at Du 16, divides again and descends on either side of
the spine to enter the Kidneys. The Governing Vessel and the
Conception Vessel are Yin and Yang projections towards the exterior of the vibrancy of Ming Men.

The ascending power of the Governing Vessel brings Yang and
spiritual stimulation to the brain. This facilitates the proper
functioning of the upper orifices of perception and the cognitive
functions that allow adaptation to the external environment.
With its numerous connections to other functions, the Governing
Vessel controls the animation of the entire body. It is sometimes
referred to as the Sea of the Yang Meridians.

The Governing Vessel is actually a mediator between the brain
and the Heart. In reading texts on Chinese Medicine and Taoist
Alchemy, Spirit is often mentioned both in reference to the Heart
and the brain. The Heart is said to "house the Spirit" and the Upper Tan Tien (brain) is called Spirit House. This linking of brain
and Heart by the Governing Vessel substantiates both views in
their proper context.

The Turtle begins with the practitioner standing with feet shoulder width and hands at the sides. He raises his hands inhaling—
bringing energy up in the body. Next the knees are slightly bent,
the upper body is leaned forward and the fists are placed on the
navel with the elbows pushed forward. With the neck extended
by tucking the chin, this position creates a strong "bowing" of the
spine. The POOH sound is made to protect the Heart.

Now the practitioner turns his head to the left with tension in
the neck while inhaling. The head is returned to straight while

holding the breath. The head is then turned to the right while inhaling and then returned to straight while holding the breath. This left/right turning is repeated for six breaths—three turns to each side. The exercise ends with a Half Basic and a Basic.

The posture itself opens the Governing Vessel. Turning the head from side to side is a common practice to stimulate the Ming Men. In this position the turning stimulates both the Ming Men and the Governing Vessel. It also activates the Lymph system in the neck.

The position of the fists brings TB 4 acupoints on each hand together thus activating them.

TB 4 is the Source Point of the Triple Burner. The Triple Burner distributes Source Chi from the Kidney/Ming Men complex to the Twelve Primary Meridians, each of which has a Source Point to receive energy from and to communicate with the Source via the Triple Burner. TB 4 is particularly used in the Japanese Acupuncture Traditions, typically with a gold needle, to strengthen Source Chi.

1.11 | DOUBLE BREATHING (TAN TIEN BREATHING)
Lower Tan Tien

THE LOWER TAN TIEN is located just below the navel. Authorities differ on its exact location and in fact the location can vary in different individuals. The perception of the location of the Lower Tan Tien can change for each individual at various stages of training. Complete Chi Kung systems will provide the tools for the student's relationship with the Lower Tan Tien to become closer and more exact as his practice matures.

The Lower Tan Tien is the foundation of the body and the root of all Taoist Practices. It is the original source of energy, both as the original area of conception and the area where sustenance enters the body from the mother via the umbilical cord. It not only stores the Original Chi (derived from parents at conception), but also acts as a storehouse where Chi from all sources is collected, blended and transformed.

The Lower Tan Tien is the underlying energetic substratum around which revolve all other energetic manifestations in the body, and is a manifestation of an even more profound universal energy. It is here that the energy of Heaven, Earth and Man interface.

The exercise begins with the practitioner standing normally with hands at the sides. The hands are raised to head level while inhaling. Next the hands are lowered in fists to the lower abdomen and the breath is "swallowed" to the Lower Tan Tien (Lower Tan Tien extends). The practitioner then inhales again. Raising the right open hand to the level of the mouth, the practitioner now makes the POOH sound to exhale the air from the second inhale (which was in the Lungs) and hisses out the air from the first inhale (which was in the Lower Tan Tien) while contracting the Lower Tan Tien.

Swallowing air (energy) to the Lower Tan Tien has been regarded as a primary means of gathering energy since ancient times. Energy gathered in the Lower Tan Tien helps blood and lymph flow thus reducing the workload for the Heart, increases hormone production, enhances digestion and elimination and allows for the storing and restoring of Chi.

In our Taoist Chi Kung, the "swallowing" technique is used more than any other technique except the Basic. Almost all the exercises past the first 18 begin with a swallow to the Lower Tan Tien. This technique both activates the deepest energies of the body and produces a hydraulic effect to increase the efficacy of whatever exercise follows.

If one were to look at Chi as money, the Lower Tan Tien would be your bank account and the Lungs would handle your pocket change.

Double Breathing begins to teach the practitioner how to differentiate his bank account from his pocket change.

YANG is related to the upper part of the body and activity. The arms are usually the vehicle for manifesting activity in the upper body and the upper arms provide power for that manifestation.

In terms of Yang energy channels, the channels of the Triple Burner, Small Intestine, and Large Intestine all traverse the arm. Located on the midline at the base of the neck below the spinous process of the seventh cervical vertebra, Governing Vessel 14 is the meeting point of all the Yang channels of the arms and legs. By filling the Yang channels of the arms through Energy to the Upper Arms, GV 14 is flushed with energy thereby either directly or indirectly activating all the Yang channels. The bent knee (horse) position assumed in this exercise "sinks" energy in the body. This activates the Yang channels of the legs because they bring energy down to the feet.

The exercise begins with the practitioner standing with feet shoulder width apart, open hands, palms facing up beside the chest. The palms are fully extended out at shoulder height with tension while inhaling. They are then turned palms downward, fists are formed and the fists are returned to the chest with tension and again inhaling. These two movements collect energy in the arms and upper body both by the tension and by the multiple inhaling. Governing Vessel 14 is also activated through the expansion and contraction of its local area, as happens throughout the exercise.

The energy from the chest is then "swallowed" to the Lower Tan Tien, both activating and strengthening the Source Chi. The POOH sound is made. Energy will be held in the Lower Tan Tien throughout the exercise. This serves to connect the power of the Lower Tan Tien to areas addressed by the exercise.

The exercise continues by alternately pushing the open palms across the chest, grabbing with the fingers and returning fists to the sides of the chest. These movements are repeated three times on each side with great tension held in the upper arms throughout. The effect is to engorge the upper arms with energy from the tension and multiple inhales while activating GV 14 through expansion and contraction.

The exercise ends with a Half Basic and a Basic.

STRATEGY NOTE | *The Yin energies of the body have been harmonized and encouraged to perform their functions of storing, categorizing, and utilizing essence. They have been linked to both the overriding intelligence and power centers of the body. The Yang energies have been brought from the depths and activated to perform their functions of collecting essence through the digestive process and defending the body.*

1.13 | DIAPHRAGM
Increases range of motion of diaphragm—digestive system

THE DIAPHRAGM is a musculomembranous wall separating the abdomen from the thoracic cavity. It convexes upward in a resting state, contracts downward upon inhalation and relaxes upward on exhalation.

In Chi Kung practices from many systems, exercises which feature one arm/shoulder raised while the other is lowered are said to strengthen the Spleen/digestive system. The usual explanation is that this position stretches the diaphragm in such a way that it massages the digestive organs. This is mechanically true. At the same time this position pumps the Urinary Bladder Channels on the back and directly stimulates the Kidneys and Ming Men—whose upward channel underlies the inner channel of the Urinary Bladder. The Ming Men is the source of digestive fire and the inner channel of the Urinary Bladder has points that nourish all the organs.

By training Diaphragm, the range of motion of the diaphragm is increased resulting not only in an abdominal organ massage but also in an increase in the amount of air inhaled and exhaled from the Lungs. An increase in the oxygen/carbon dioxide exchange vitalizes and cleans the body as a whole.

The exercise begins with feet less than shoulder width and hands at the sides. The open hands are raised to the level of the head while inhaling, then dropped to the lower abdomen with hands in fists. The POOH sound is made and the fists are placed at the sides of the legs. From this position the left shoulder is raised and the right shoulder is lowered while inhaling. Next the right shoulder is raised while the left shoulder is lowered while exhaling. This raising and lowering motion coordinated with inhaling and exhaling is performed 12 times. The exercise ends with a Basic. Then the whole process is repeated on the opposite side—raising the right shoulder first while inhaling, etc.

1.14 | THYROID
Thyroid Gland

THE THYROID GLAND originates from the same area and, in fact, the same tissue as the anterior lobe of the Pituitary gland. It is an energy producing gland, influencing metabolism, growth, and the stamina of the whole body. The Thyroid helps build brain and nervous tissue and is a link between the brain and the sexual organs. Sexual arousal, menstruation, and pregnancy directly affect the Thyroid. In the evolutionary past, this gland allowed certain sea animals to dwell on land. It controls our speed of living. Thyroid secretion stimulates gastric peristalsis and all metabolic processes while aiding in the detoxification of the body.

The throat is related to communication—speech. In Chinese Medicine, the tongue is related to the Heart—mind. Smooth energy flow between Heart and tongue facilitate clear communications.

This area is said to be related to "possession" by external entities. Because speech is so closely related to breath and of course breath is closely related to Chi, the area has an unusually direct link with our energy body. In theory, if the practitioner is training a balanced system, he should be protected at each level of development.

Some styles of Taoist Chi Kung practice dream work, and meditation on the throat area is one of the techniques used to consciously cross from the waking to the dream state. The Chi Kung we are concerned with here does not practice dream work although there are other sleep related techniques in Level 2. Our system believes your mind should be quiet when you sleep—thus dream-less.

The exercise begins with the practitioner standing normally with hands at the sides. He raises his open hands to head level while inhaling and drops them to the lower abdomen forming fists and making the POOH sound. From there the fists are moved to the sides of the thighs with the palm side facing the body. The practitioner then rotates his fists backward until the backs of the fists touch the thigh. At the same time he tightens his jaw, neck and arms and pushes down with the fists. Next he relaxes. The tightening—relaxing technique is repeated 24 times while breathing normally. The exercise ends with a Basic.

This exercise engorges the neck and Yang channels of the arms with energy. The Yang channels of the arms directly influence the neck, thus the Thyroid Gland.

The Lymphatic System in the neck is also activated during this exercise. The Thyroid can work miracles if done at the first sign of a sore throat (add several Tigers and Energy Escape from the Skin for good measure).

1.15 | NOSE

Yang Ming (Large Intestine and Stomach); Ming Men

TAOISTS BELIEVE that the nose is directly related to the Ming Men. This exercise brings attention to the tip of the nose thus activates Ming Men. In Nose, the Large Intestine channel is activated by the hand positions and the Stomach is activated by the stance. Both the Larger Intestine and the Stomach are indispensable in the digestive process which leads to generation of Chi and absorption of Essences.

In Chinese Medicine, the Large Intestine is in charge of separating the clear from the turbid. The turbid is excreted as feces and the clear reabsorbed by the body. Parts of this reabsorbed material are essences which were not absorbed by the Spleen. These essences are transported to the Kidneys to fuel the Ming Men fire, source of Kidney Yang which is the root of digestive energy.

The Lung is also activated in this exercise. With Metal being the generator of Water, both Kidney Yin and Yang are nourished through the Nose.

The exercise begins with the practitioner standing with feet wide apart, hands at sides. The hands are raised to the level of the head while inhaling and dropped to the lower abdomen in fists. The POOH sound is made. The practitioner then leans to the left while placing the left hand on the waist, straightening the right leg and bending the left. This position engorges the Yang channels of the body, especially the Stomach. It particularly activates ST 36 which is known as the most important acupoint on the body to stimulate the generation of Chi and Blood by the Spleen/Stomach. It is an important point to harmonize the Stomach, strengthen the Spleen, resolve dampness, strengthen Yang, clear fire and calm the Spirit.

The practitioner then extends the first and middle fingers and brings the thumb to meet the curled ring and little finger on the right hand. While inhaling he raises the right hand to the left shoulder—stimulating the Lung at LU 1 at the shoulder. He then stretches his arm in a large 180° arc to the right side while exhaling. The arm is returned along the same arc until the right hand is once again at the left shoulder. The two outstretched fingertips remain pointed upwards throughout the movements. The Large Intestine channel runs from the bottom corner of the fingernail of the first finger, up the arm and neck and ends at the nose. This arm movement engorges that channel with energy. The arm movement with coordinated breathing is repeated 12 times and the exercise ends with a Basic. The whole process is repeated on the left side.

1.16 | RUBBING THE STOMACH, INTESTINES & GALL BLADDER
Digestive System

THIS EXERCISE acts primarily on the three acupoints CV 12, GB 24, and Liv 14.

CV 12, known as Middle Cavity or Middle Controller, is the meeting point for the energy of all the Yang Organs. Traditionally it is said to treat all diseases of the Stomach and Spleen. It is one of the primary points used for treating digestive problems caused from emotional issues. CV 12 is another point used to strengthen overall Yang in the body.

This point is also believed to control the body's external energy field. Thoughts and emotions affect our external energy field and if this point is out of balance and in contact with other such fields one can be adversely affected by others' mental and emotional states.

CV 12 marks the center of the Middle Cauldron where Fire energy from the Middle Tan Tien and Water energy from the Lower Tan Tien are mixed in Level 2 training.

GB 24, known as Sun and Moon, is the point on the front of the body where the energy of the Gall Bladder gathers. It is used to treat dysfunction of the Gall Bladder itself and problems affecting the Gall bladder from such causes as emotional disharmony and disharmony in the Stomach or Spleen.

LIV 14, known as Cycle Gate, is the point on the front of the body where the energy of the Liver gathers. It harmonizes blood and energy flow in the Upper and Middle Burners, harmonizes Liver and Stomach, and spreads Liver Chi.

All three of these points clear stagnation and keep things moving smoothly in the digestive system.

The exercise begins with the practitioner standing normally with hands at the sides. He raises his hands to head level while inhaling and drops the fists to the lower abdomen. The POOH sound is made.

Bending at the waist, the right hand is placed on the right side above the navel and the left hand is placed on top of the right. Both hands are then rubbed to the left side while inhaling and returned to the right side exhaling. This cycle is repeated 9 times. The exercise ends with a Basic. The process is then repeated on the left side. The rubbing is done with enough friction to generate heat. Aside from stimulating the three points mentioned above, the exercise warms the upper abdomen and does stimulate other points that help digestion. The bending at the waist stimulates the Ming Men.

1.17 | ENERGY TO THE SOLES
Yang Leg Channels, Connection to the Earth

The Yang channels of the legs carry energy from the body to the feet. The only acupoint on the sole of the foot is KI 1. KI 1, referred to as Gushing Spring or Earth Surge, is the place where the energies of Earth and Man conjoin. It is an important point in balancing the body and absorbing energy from the Earth to supplement the body's own energy.

Energy to the Soles engorges the legs with Chi, extending that energy into the Earth. When the exercise ends, a backlash of both the body's energy and energy from the Earth rushes into the body to nourish our energy and increase overall circulation.

The exercise begins with the practitioner standing with hands at the sides and feet close together with the toes pointed slightly inwards. The hands are raised to the level of the head while inhaling. They are then dropped to the lower abdomen in fists while swallowing energy to the Lower Tan Tien. The POOH sound is made.

Next the open palms are raised to the level of the chest while inhaling again. The fists are pushed down to the lower abdomen while the knees bend. While looking down, squeezing the toes and tightening the legs, energy is pushed from the Lower Tan Tien to

the feet. This position is held as long as comfortable. The exercise
ends with a Half Basic and a Basic.

STRATEGY NOTE | *With the Diaphragm we have massaged
the digestive system and activated Ming Men. The Thyroid stimulates the metabolism and the Nose adds fuel to the digestive fire.
Rubbing the Stomach, Intestines and Gall Bladder invigorates the
digestive system and removes obstructions, and Energy to the
Soles facilitates absorption of energy from the earth as well as
activating the Yang leg channels. By this time in the system we
have activated all the organs for essence gathering and essence
matriculation.*

1.18 | STRENGTHEN THE ABDOMINAL REGION
Lower Tan Tien

THE LOWER TAN TIEN has already been discussed. This
exercise is interesting because it uses external vibration to
stimulate development. When the Lower Tan Tien is "filled" with
energy from sitting practices—or other techniques—it will spontaneously begin to vibrate. The vibration is a result of "filling" and
will generate even more energy. The energy then spills out into the
channels to invigorate the body. This exercise attempts to artifi-
cially vibrate the Lower Tan Tien for the same ends. One interesting aspect of the exercise position is that by holding the toes
upright, energy from the legs will flow upwards to concentrate in
the Lower Tan Tien. This of course uses the previous Leg exercise
to add to the efficacy of Strengthen the Abdominal Region. Holding the legs and torso up will also exercise the abdominal muscles.

The exercise begins with the practitioner sitting on the floor or in a
backless chair. He raises his open hands to head level and inhales,
then drops the hands in fists to the lower abdomen while swallowing energy to the Lower Tan Tien. Next he raises his legs with toes
flexed up and leans backwards balancing on his buttocks. While
breathing normally from the Lungs but holding energy in the Lower Tan Tien he strikes the fists of both hands on the abdomen just

below the navel 24 times. To end the exercise he returns to sitting while doing a Half Basic and then stands to do a Basic. Each day one more hit is added until he is doing a total of 48 each time.

STRATEGY NOTE | *One of the classics of Chinese Medicine states that the body has "Four Seas" and twelve meridians that are like rivers that flow into the "Seas." The "Seas are specialized energy systems that support basic functions of the body/mind/Spirit complex.*

- The **Sea of Nourishment** supports digestive function.

- The **Sea of Marrow** supports brain function.

- The **Sea of Chi** supports rhythms and movement in the body.

- The **Sea of Blood** (Chong Mai) supports dissemination of essences through blood circulation.

The exercises relating to digestion tonify the Sea of Nourishment. Whenever the legs are bent one of its main access points (ST 36) is activated. The other "Seas" will be addresses in the next section of exercises.

1.19 | ENERGY TO THE UPPER BACK
Defensive Energy, Immune System

THERE are two important functions for this exercise, and four acupoints utilized to accomplish these functions.

The first function is to strengthen the body's ability to resist external illness. In Chinese Medicine, it is believed that external illnesses are predisposed to enter the body from the upper back and neck, especially near GV 14.

The second function is to open the channels of energetic communication between the Source energy and the upper body both for strengthening defensive energy and for making extra energy available to manifest in the upper body as needed.
As we have already mentioned, GV 14 is the meeting place of all

six Yang vessels of the hand and the six Yang vessels of the foot. As external diseases penetrate from the outside (Yang) towards the inside, this point is well suited to address external problems. GV 14 is not only able to expel external pathogens, but also able to tonify our defensive energy. Owing to its ability to control the pores, dispel pathogenic heat, and tonify deficiency, GV 14 is a major point in regulating the body's sweating. As one of the points directly relating to the Sea of Chi, GV 14 can also treat deficiency and exhaustion of the whole body and painful obstructions anywhere in the body. GV 14 also affects the whole spinal column.

UB 11 is a point that is also very influential in activating the defense mechanisms of the body. It also is the "meeting place of the bones" and is used to address any problems with bones. As the Kidneys "control the bones," UB 11 is closely associated with the Kidneys. Our system of Chi Kung makes extensive use of this connection to the Kidneys and bones (especially the spine) in several exercises.

UB 11 is also directly related to the "Sea of Blood." Chong Mai is referred to as the Sea of Blood and this point accesses that "Sea." This makes a point that can increase blood flow—thus essence distribution. In later levels Chong Mai is extensively used for transporting refined energy to feed the Spirit.

STRATEGY NOTE | *It is interesting to note that the above two points address the external part of the body via the Yang channels and also the depths of the body via the bones.*

TB 4 is the Source Point of the Triple Burner. The Triple Burner distributes Source Chi from the Kidney/Ming Men complex to the Twelve Primary Meridians, each of which has a Source Point to receive energy from and to communicate with the Source via the Triple Burner. TB 4 is particularly used in the Japanese Acupuncture Traditions, typically with a gold needle, to strengthen Source Chi.

The overall exercise strengthens and activates the deep energies to support the defensive capability of the body, open channels of communication for physical manifestation of energy in the upper body and to increase blood circulation (external attacks can deplete blood leading to painful obstructions) especially in the upper body.

The exercise begins with the practitioner standing with feet shoulder width and hands at the sides. He raises his hands to the level of the head while inhaling and lowers his fists to the Lower Tan Tien while swallowing and making the POOH sound. Next he bends his knees and brings his hands together (back to back) in the front of his body. The arms push down to spread the upper back, the tailbone and chin tuck to open the spine, and the legs bend to pull energy from the upper body down. This position opens and empties the upper back.

Now the practitioner contracts his Lower Tan Tien and does a long slow inhale directing the energy to the upper back. The exercise ends with a Half Basic and a Basic.

1.20 | ENERGY TO 2 SIDES
External trauma, Sea of Chi

ENERGY TO TWO SIDES works through vibrating the chest cavity, Gall Bladder Channel and activating two principal acupoints.

SP 21, known as the Great Envelope, is an acupoint that influences the blood of all the connecting channels of the body. These channels function to distribute Chi and especially blood to all the tissues of the body. From this point the tissues of the whole body can be affected. SP 21 not only regulates the Chi and Blood but also strengthens the sinews and joints. Many systems of Chi Kung utilize training this point to strengthen the body's resistance to external trauma and facilitate speedy healing.

GB 23 known as Flank Sinews, is a point that regulates the Chi in the Three Burners. It is also used for releasing symptoms from unexpressed anger, frustration, and resentment—which may well accompany physical trauma as well as come from other causes. In some traditions this point is accepted as the front meeting point of the Gall Bladder, which gives it great influence on the Gall Bladder energy.

Energy to Two Sides stretches the Gall Bladder Meridian by body position, and strongly activates it through the vibrations caused by pounding the sides. The Gall Bladder Meridian begins near the outer canthus of the eye and ends on the lateral side of the tip of the fourth toe (bilateral). It traverses the entire side of the body. The sides of the body are areas where Yin and Yang meet. The Gall Bladder is sometimes referred to as a hinge linking the inside and outside—Yin and Yang. The activation of the channel can have a balancing effect on the whole body. The Gall Bladder is also influential in problems with the body's articulations.

The point of departure for the Chi of the entire body is the Sea of Chi, located in the chest and activated by this exercise. The Sea of Chi, through its connection with the Heart, spreads energy throughout the body. The Heart, in charge of the channels and circulation of blood is also stimulated by Energy to the Two Sides. With the Lungs (also activated by the vibrations in the chest) governing the rhythm of the Chi, and the Heart governing the blood, this exercise has a powerful effect of balancing and rebalancing both Chi and Blood in the body.

The exercise begins with the practitioner standing with feet wide apart. He raises his hands to the level of the head while inhaling, drops his fists to the lower abdomen while swallowing to the Lower Tan Tien, and makes the POOH sound.

He then leans to the right, stretching out his left leg and bending his right leg. At the same time he raises his left elbow and inhales. Next he swings his right fist forcefully up to connect with his left side under the armpit. This "thumping" is repeated five times. The practitioner then does a Half Basic and a Basic to complete the first half of the exercise. The whole process is repeated on the right side.

1.21 | EAR EXERCISE
Sea of Marrow

MANY STYLES of Chi Kung contain a variation of this exercise. Usually called "Beating the Heavenly Drum," the Ear exercise is said to clear the mind and consolidate the Spirit. This result is attributed to stimulating the area of the acupoint GV 16, known as Palace of Wind for its ability to expel pathogenic wind factors of both external and internal origin. Being one of the points that directly accesses the Sea of Marrow, GV 16 also has the ability to nourish the brain. It is a meeting point of the Governing Vessel and Yang Linking Vessel, which extends its realm of influence beyond its local region. The Governing Vessel enters the brain at GV 16, with another branch reaching the Heart. With the Heart "controlling the Spirit" and the brain being the residence of the Original Spirit, it is easy to see how the point can affect mind and Spirit.

There is another aspect of this exercise that is seldom mentioned. It is true that GV 16 is activated during the Ear, but the index finger containing the beginning of the Large Intestine Channel is also strongly stimulated. This activates the channel which in turn stimulates the organ.

Remember it is the Large Intestine that separates the "clear from the turbid" in the Lower Burner. The turbid is excreted and the clear is reabsorbed to fuel the fire of Ming Men. This generates more activity in Ming Men, resulting in increased defensive energy production and a rising of the pure Yang to the head to clear the brain and consolidate the Spirit.

The exercise begins with the practitioner standing normally with hands at the sides. He raises his hands to the level of the head while inhaling, then lowers his fists to the lower abdomen while swallowing. The POOH sound is made.

The palms are then clasped tightly over the ears with the fingers wrapping around the head towards the rear. The index finger is "snapped" sharply off the middle finger onto the area around GV 16 seventy two times while breathing normally. Some traditions prefer to have only the two fingers in use to touch the head as the other fingers may "blunt" the vibrations. Some traditions keep the elbows pointed to the sides, while our tradition has the elbows pointed forward to encourage the vibration to travel from the rear Pituitary Gland to the forward Pineal Gland. The exercise ends with a Basic.

1.22 | MOVING THE ENERGY UP AND DOWN
The Chi Mechanism

MOVING the Energy Up and Down addresses the same areas as the Diaphragm, but gives greater emphasis to the actual ascending and descending energies that characterize the digestive system.

Chi Mechanism is a term used to reflect the proper functioning of the Stomach/Spleen in "raising the pure" and "downbearing the turbid."

The Stomach is in charge of "rotting and ripening"—the initial stages of digestion. The energy of the Stomach is descending in nature, moving waste through the bowels.

The Spleen is in charge of "transformation and transportation"— extracting the finest essences from food and transporting them upwards to the Lung where they mix with oxygen to form blood. The blood moves to the Heart (where it acquires its red color—the mark of the Spirits) and is propelled throughout the body.

If the Spleen fails to move the pure essences upward the pure can be discharged through the bowels resulting in malnutrition. If the Spleen fails to extract the essences and the Stomach fails to properly descend waste, the turbid may pollute the newly formed blood.

Complications from improper "raising the pure" and "downbearing the turbid" can cause dampness to descend to the lower burner resulting in damp heat or Chi stagnation. Both conditions can disrupt the fire of Ming Men which in turn will disrupt other organ functions. The disruption of Ming Men fire causes a wide variety of symptoms, often difficult to diagnose and treat.

The exercise begins with the palm side of right fist over the palm side of the left fist at the level of the navel. The right fist is raised overhead and the left fist is lowered to the left side while inhaling. The inhale is swallowed to the Lower Tan Tien and the POOH sound is made. The left fist is then raised overhead and the right fist lowered to the right side while inhaling. The practitioner then exhales through his nose. He then inhales again and swallows to the lower Tan Tien, followed by the POOH. Again he changes hands—lowering the left to the left side and raising the right overhead while inhaling. He then exhales through the nose. The hands are returned to the starting position while inhaling. The exercise is completed with a Half Basic and a Basic.

The raising and lowering of the hands combined with multiple inhales and "swallows" links the ascending and descending energies to the center and fortifies their directions and pathways.

1.23 | LEG EXERCISE
Leg and Connection to the Earth.

THIS EXERCISE is a more intense version of Energy to the Soles. It utilizes Chi Packing techniques to fully engorge the legs with energy.

The practitioner begins by bending the left knee and extending the right leg to the side with toes pointed up. The position of the extended leg pushes energy up to the Lower Tan Tien and from there into the left leg to increase energy flow to that leg.

The practitioner then raises his hands to the level of the head while inhaling, drops his fists to the lower abdomen while swallowing energy to the Lower Tan Tien and then makes the POOH sound. He raises his open palms to the chest while inhaling and pushes his fists down over the left leg, forcing energy into the leg. After holding that position for a short time, he again raises his palms to the chest—no inhale—and pushes his fists down over the left leg again forcing energy into the leg. The raising the palms and lowering fists motion is performed one more time. In this process, the mind is used to engorge the leg with energy.

The exercise ends with a Half Basic and a Basic, and is then repeated on the other side.

STRATEGY NOTE | *Reflecting basic Yin/Yang theory, it is often accepted that opposites support and reflect each other. In the previous exercise, the energy of the body was concentrated in the feet. In the next exercise energy will be concentrated in the top of the body. The feet, as we shall see in later explorations, are intimately connected to the head through several avenues including the Kidney Channel and the Chong Mai which both have a presence on the sole.*

1.24 | BODY STAND ON SHOULDERS
Digestive Organs, Circulation in Upper Body

IN CHINESE MEDICINE the Spleen is said to control the function of "holding the organs in place" with its uplifting energy. Body Stand on Shoulders places the body in an inverted position, reversing the effect of gravity on the internal organs and supporting the Spleen's upholding function. This position obviously enhances blood flow to the upper body as well, bringing more essences to the brain.

The exercise begins with the practitioner seated on the ground. He raises his hands while inhaling and lowers his fists to the thighs while swallowing energy to the Lower Tan Tien and following with the POOH sound. The next step is to roll backwards to a regular shoulder stand with hands supporting the hips—elbows on the floor.

When the legs are straight up and the position is stable, the legs are spread sideways to a medium width and the hissing sound of the Liver is made. This is to relieve excess pressure in the upper body and expel toxin. The legs are brought together again and the position is held for from two to five minutes. It may be held longer. Every twenty or thirty seconds or whenever excess pressure is felt the leg spreading/hissing action is performed, followed by a return to the upright position.

To end the exercise, the practitioner lowers himself to the sitting position and does a Half Basic. He then stands and does a Basic.

1.25 | FACIAL MASSAGE
Clear the Spirit, Invigorate the Yang Channels

THE THREE YANG CHANNELS of the arms and three Yang Channels of the legs all either begin or end on the face. The face itself contains micro systems of acupoints that affect the whole body. Stimulation of the face invigorates these channels and systems.

Spiritual energy is said to express itself in the face, as the "brightness of the Spirits." By invigorating the energy of the face, the Spirit can be "brightened" or cleaned.

The exercise begins with the practitioner standing normally. He raises his hands to the level of the head while inhaling, drops his fists to the lower abdomen while swallowing energy to the Lower Tan Tien and then makes the POOH sound.

Placing the right fingertips on the right side of the chin, he rubs across his forehead with his left palm thirty six times. Next he places the index fingers of both hands on the outer canthus and the middle fingers of both hands on the inner canthus, and rubs up and down eighteen times. This is followed by placing the thumbs of both hands behind the ears with the palms on the cheeks and rubbing another eighteen times. Finally the right fingertips are again placed on the right side of the chin and the left hand is rubbed across the entire face horizontally thirty six times. The exercise ends with a Basic. The practitioner breaths normally during the exercise.

1.26 | EIGHT WAYS OF TAI CHI BREATHING
Eight Extra-OrdinaryVessels

THE EIGHT Extra-Ordinary Meridians are vital aspects of our most primitive constitution. They are the initial organizers of those forces that will produce our being and remain fundamental distributors of Essence, Chi and Spirit throughout our lives. They represent the organizational parameters of the body, controlling the powers that create and balance our personal manifestation of the union of energies that precede our form. The Eight Extra-Ordinary Meridians organize the original Yin and Yang of our bodies.

The Eight Extra-Ordinary Meridians are often viewed as reservoirs of energy for the rest of the body, accepting excess energy from the system and releasing energy to deficient areas. They preserve normal functioning of the body at the deepest levels.

The Governing Vessel expresses Chi and Yang at the deepest level. The Conception Vessel expresses Blood and Yin. Chong Mai is the bursting forth of life from the original Yin and Yang, while Dai Mai provides boundaries for that life. Yin and Yang Chiao Mai regulate the rhythms and interpenetration of Yin and Yang, while Yin and Yang Wei Mai organize the systems of Blood and Yin and Chi and Yang. From these original organizations spring the functional responsibilities of the Twelve Regular Meridians and their Organs.

This exercise is the most physically complicated one in the system. When my teacher taught me Eight Ways of Tai Chi Breathing he said it could bring "unlimited power." At that time I remembered that many years previous to my introduction to Chi Kung, I had read about a Taoist Technique that was believed to develop unlimited power—but the technique was lost. If this was the same technique, it had evidently survived in our oral tradition. This exercise was also the precursor to Tai Chi Chuan according to my teacher.

The exercise begins with the practitioner standing with feet moderately wide apart and hands at the sides. The open palms are raised to the navel with the right hand on top of the left while gently inhaling. This movement opens the body to the energies from Earth through the feet and perineum. Next the hands are dropped to the sides while gently exhaling—returning the gathered Earth energy while keeping the connection open. The open palms are then raised up and to the sides until overhead while inhaling—connecting Earth Energy to Heaven Energy through the practitioner. The five fingertips are brought together—consolidating the energies of the Five Elements in man with the joined energies of Heaven and Earth—this is interesting in that it links the primal energies of Heaven and Earth which exist before the Eight Extra-Ordinary Vessels with the Five Elemental Energies which form in man after the Eight Extra-Ordinary Vessels (prenatal and postnatal energies). The hands are then lowered down the centerline of the body to the ground while gently exhaling, to consolidate the union of Heaven, Earth, and Man.

What follows are twelve vigorous inhales coordinated with fairly forceful body movements. Each movement is designed to activate one of the Eight Extra-Ordinary Vessels. There are twelve breaths and movements because the movements for Yin and Yang Chiao and Yin and Yang Wei are performed bi-laterally. The Chong Mai movement is performed twice to emphasize its function of vigorously upthrusting life energy and the Governing Vessel and Conception Vessel are linked together in one movement to consolidate the basic Yin/Yang co-penetration that is a prerequisite for being.

The two Chong Mai motions are thrusting motions up the midline of the body including squatting. The four motions for Yin and Yang Chiao Mai involve lunges and retractions of the feet to the sides with accompanying arm pushes and retractions. The two Yin Wei movements involve pulling energy down from overhead to the legs on both sides of the body and the two Yang Wei motions involve outward circling and returning of the arms at chest level. The Governing Vessel and Conception Vessel are addressed by a wide outward and uprising vertical circling of the arms overhead and returning them to the front of the body down the centerline. Dai Mai is activated by circling the hands from the Lower Tan Tien out to the sides, forward and straight back in to the Lower Tan Tien. The exercise ends with a Half Basic and a Basic.

STRATEGY NOTE | *After activating all Eight Extra-Ordinary Vessels, the following exercise stimulates and balances the rhythms of Blood and Chi flow throughout the body by activating the Sea of Chi.*

1.27 | SIDE HITTING STYLE
Defensive Energy, Sea of Chi

THIS EXERCISE basically addresses the same areas as Energy to Two Sides but with a different emphasis. In Energy to Two Sides the vibrations from the pounding activated the Gall Bladder Channel and penetrated through the whole chest cavity. Side Hitting Style does not activate the Gall Bladder Meridian as strongly and the vibrations penetrate from both sides at once to create a more intense stimulation of the Sea of Chi.

The exercise begins with the practitioner standing with feet moderately wide apart and the hands at the sides. As in the Hawk, he raises his fists forward and outward at chest level while inhaling. Next he forcefully slaps both upper arms onto the sides of the body and exhales sharply, then bends forward and thrusts his fists straight down exhaling forcefully again. These double exhales are used to protect the Heart and Lungs from the meeting of the powerful energy waves produced by the slapping of the arms on the sides. The exercise ends with a Basic.

The whole process is repeated two more times for a total of three repetitions.

1.28 | THREE BREATHS OF ENERGY
Invigorate Body

TAN TIEN BREATHING (Double Breathing), Three Breaths of Energy, Four Breathing and Five Breathing comprise a group of exercises designed to move large amounts of energy to various important areas of the body. Beginning with Tan Tien Breathing, these exercises build on their predecessors to develop sophisticated methods of moving and controlling energy in the body. In the process, they invigorate the entire body and, as we shall see in later discussions, support and balance the Five Element energies.

The exercise begins with the practitioner standing normally with hands at the sides. He raises his hands to the level of the head while inhaling, then drops his fists to the lower abdomen as he swallows energy to the Lower Tan Tien.

The energy held in the Lower Tan Tien is then moved to the upper back by assuming an abbreviated Energy to the Upper Back posture while sucking in the Lower Tan Tien and consciously directing the energy to the expanded upper back.

Another inhale is swallowed to the Lower Tan Tien, followed by an inhale to the Lungs. At this point the practitioner is holding energy in his upper back, Lower Tan Tien, and Lungs.

The POOH sound is made to expel energy from the Lungs. The Lower Tan Tien is contracted and the energy held there is hissed out the mouth. Next, the energy held in the upper back is transferred to the Lower Tan Tien—thus expanding that area. The Lower Tan Tien is then contracted again and the energy held there (transferred from the upper back) is hissed out the mouth. The exercise concludes with a Basic.

1.29 | ENERGY ESCAPE FROM THE SKIN
Cleanse the body, expel external pathogens

THIS EXERCISE is designed to allow energy to literally escape through the skin. There are two main advantages to developing this ability.

First, external pathogens attack through the skin, so this exercise is useful in eliminating them. It is a good idea to perform this exercise at the first sign of a cold or flu—along with the Tiger and the Thyroid.

Second, when performing exercises with multiple inhales, if the practitioner has developed these energetic pathways, old, stagnant Chi will be pushed out from the inside through the infusion of clean fresh energy.

This cleanses and refreshes the body.

The exercise begins with the practitioner standing normally with hands at the sides. He raises his hands to the level of the head while inhaling, and then drops his fists to the lower abdomen as he swallows energy to the Lower Tan Tien.

The energy held in the Lower Tan Tien is then moved to the upper back by assuming an abbreviated Energy to the Upper Back posture while sucking in the Lower Tan Tien and consciously directing the energy to the expanded upper back.

Another inhale is swallowed to the Lower Tan Tien, followed by an inhale to the Lungs. At this point the practitioner is holding energy in his upper back, Lower Tan Tien, and Lungs.

To allow the Lung energy to escape from the chest, three large outward swinging arm movements are performed. To allow the energy held in the Lower Tan Tien to escape, the fists are held at the sides level with the Lower Tan Tien and pushed out and returned three times while expanding and contracting the Lower Tan Tien and slightly raising and dipping the knees. To allow the energy held in the upper back to escape, the arms are held in the Monkey position (from Monkey exercise), and the shoulders are rolled forwards and backwards—expanding and relaxing the upper back. Any remaining energy is swallowed to the Tan Tien, the assumption being that by this time the practitioner is swallowing fresh, clean energy and has pushed out the old.

The practitioner's goal is to be able to perform this whole technique nine times without having to exhale. Of course this level of expertise takes a long time to develop.

The exercise ends with a Basic—usually it ends with the practitioner blurting out a Half Basic from all the energy that did not escape from his skin, and then a Basic. : >)

1.30 | TENDON AND LIGAMENT EXERCISE
Physical Form

TRADITIONALLY Tendon and Ligament type exercises are used to train our physical form including the muscles, tendons, ligaments, bones and fasciae. The form must be kept healthy to support the energy for Spiritual evolvement. Aside from strengthening the physical body, these exercises develop defensive energy and eliminate stagnation.

Although Tendon and Ligament Exercise does not specifically target the internal organs (except the Liver), it will have a powerful effect on them. All the body's internal organs have areas at the level of the musculature that they directly relate to via their channels. After engorging those areas with Chi during the tension phase of the exercises, a flood of Chi will flow back to the organs when the tension is released. This invigorates and removes stagnation both externally and internally.

The Liver is said to control the tendons and ligaments of the whole body, thus the exercises will have a special effect on that energy system.

It is interesting to note that after a long time of practicing the Tendon and Ligament Exercise, the practitioner will feel the energy reach all the way to the bones. After a considerably longer time, energy that penetrated to the depths of the bones will actually expand outward through the skin. These exercises have a much greater range of activity than the superficial layers of the body.

"The connective tissues are an amazingly plastic, malleable, changeable, and highly functional group of tissues. That the classical Chinese authors related the Triple Warmer and the conduction of Chi to the fascia and their connective tissues well before scientific measurement was able to demonstrate such activity is a remarkable achievement." (from *Hara Diagnosis: Reflections on the Sea* by Kiko Matsumoto and Steven Birch, page 163—Paradigm Publications 1988).

"Oschman summarizes the basic physiological model of these structures quite elegantly: The connective tissue and fascia form a mechanical continuum, extending throughout the animal body, even to the innermost parts of each cell. All great systems of the body—the circulation, the nervous system, the musculo-skeletal system, the digestive tract, the various organs—are ensheathed in connective tissue. This matrix determines the overall shape of the organism as well as the detailed architecture of its parts. All movements, of the body as a whole, or of its smallest parts, are created by tensions carried through the connective tissue fabric. Each tension, each compression, each movement causes the crystalline lattices of the connective tissues to generate bioelectric signals that are precisely characteristic of those tensions, compressions, and movements. The fabric is a semi-conducting communication network that can convey the bioelectric signals between every part of the body and every other part. This communication network within the fascia is none other than the meridian system of Oriental Medicine, with its countless extensions into every part of the body. As these signals flow through the tissues, their biomagnetic counterparts extend the stories they tell into the space around the body. The mechanical, bioelectric, and biomagnetic signals traveling through the connective tissue, and through space around the body, tell the various cells how to form and reform the tissue architecture in response to tensions, compressions, and movements we make." (from *Hara Diagnosis: Reflections on the Sea* by Kiko Matsumoto and Steven Birch, pg. 164—Paradigm Publications 1988 (in the above quote) James Oschman, *Natural Science of Healing*, op. cit.)

These two quotes point out the enormous importance of the "Tendons and Ligaments."

The exercise begins with the practitioner standing with feet shoulder width, arms at sides. He raises his arms to the level of the head while inhaling, drops fists to the sides while swallowing energy to the Lower Tan Tien and makes the POOH sound.

While holding energy in the Lower Tan Tien and forming his hands into "special fists," he extends his arms straight out forward from the shoulders. Then he tenses his whole body and relaxes twelve times—without breathing. The exercise ends with a Half Basic and a Basic. This position tends to bring the attention of the exercise slightly to the Middle Tan Tien—Pericardium area.

Again the practitioner begins the exercise. This time, after reaching the "special fist" stage he bends forward at 90° and extends his arms backward parallel to the ground. He tenses his whole body and relaxes twelve times—without breathing. The exercise ends with a Half Basic and a Basic. This position tends to bring the attention of the exercise to the Lower Tan Tien—Kidney/Ming Men area.

For a third time he performs the beginning sequence up to the "special fist" position. This time he puts his fists together in front of the chest and tenses his whole body and relaxes twelve times—without breathing but as before holding energy in the Lower Tan Tien. The exercise ends with a Half Basic and a Basic. This position evenly distributes the effects throughout the body.

This set of exercises is the most physically challenging in the entire system.

STRATEGY NOTE | *The previous exercise, due to the physical exertion, produces appreciable waste products in the system, as well as stirring up old toxins. The next exercise is the master exercise for removing toxins from the body.*

1.31 | RIDDING THE ABDOMEN OF CARBON DIOXIDE
Cleansing the Body

IN THIS EXERCISE multiple inhales are used to widen all the channels of the body and cleansing sound is used to expel toxins. The inhaling is accomplished through the Lungs, but the bringing the energy down in the body is the function of the Kidneys. Because this energy must pass through the abdomen in its journey from Lung to Kidney, the abdomen is especially "stirred up" and cleansed. The name of the exercise reflects this situation even though toxin from the whole body is eliminated.

The exercise is performed exactly the same as the Hawk, except there are twelve inhales rather than six. Instead of the Half Basic that follows the inhales in the Hawk, the practitioner performs a slow Half Basic while squatting down low to the ground and making the hissing—cleansing sound of the Monkey. This is followed by a Basic.

1.32 | ENERGY FLOW TO KIDNEY
Strengthen Kidneys

This exercise uses body position, breath, and mind to tonify the Kidneys.

The exercise begins with the practitioner standing with feet shoulder width and hands at the sides. He inhales while lifting the hands to the level of the head and then lowers the fists to the lower abdomen while swallowing energy to the Lower Tan Tien. The POOH sound is then made.

Next the knees are bent, the hands are dropped towards the knees, the spine is bowed outward while the hips are tucked under, and the head is pulled back as far as is comfortable. The practitioner does a long, slow inhale directing the energy to the Kidneys. The head is pulled back to limit the upward motion of energy, which should gravitate towards the bowed spine at the level of the Kidneys.

The exercise ends with a Half Basic followed by the Basic.

STRATEGY NOTE | *In the above exercise, energy is collected in the Kidneys. The Hungry Tiger Catches the Lamb exercises the back, legs, and Kidneys in such a way that energy and Jing are circulated throughout the body.*

1.33 | HUNGRY TIGER CATCHING THE LAMB
Kidneys, Back and Legs, Overall Circulation

THIS EXERCISE mechanically exercises the back and legs to energize the Kidneys. The waist twisting and weight shifting strongly influence the Kidneys. The wide sweeping arm movements activate circulation throughout the body, and the Tiger Hand position opens the chest and links the circulatory system to the physical movements. In fact, energetically, the Fire from the chest and the Water from the lower abdomen mix throughout the exercise.

The exercise begins with the feet wide apart and the hands at the sides. The hands are raised to the level of the head while inhaling and the fists are dropped to the lower abdomen while swallowing energy to the Lower Tan Tien. POOH.

The weight is shifted to the right, with the right leg bending and the left leg straightening with toes pointed upwards. Tiger Hands are formed. The arms are swung in a wide arc, first to the rear and overhead and then to the ground in front—coordinated with a lunge onto the left leg and a straightening of the right leg. The practitioner inhales throughout this movement.

From this lunged to the left position the arms are again swung to the rear and up while shifting back to the weighted right leg, and continue around to the ground—again in front of a left lunge while inhaling. This technique is repeated one more time.

The exercise ends with a Half Basic and a Basic, and is then repeated on the other side.

STRATEGY NOTE | In the next exercise—Heating the Life Door, everything is consolidated to activate the Ming Men.

1.34 | HEATING THE LIFE DOOR
Ming Men

THE MING MEN has already been covered in detail. In this exercise, the Yin energies from the front of the body and the Yang energies from the back are brought together. This merging of Yin and Yang generates a 'spark' that creates heat in the Ming Men. Heating the Ming Men activates its functions.

The exercise begins with the practitioner standing with feet shoulder width apart and arms at the sides. He raises his hands to the level of the head while inhaling and drops his fists to the lower abdomen while swallowing energy to the Lower Tan Tien. The POOH sound is made.

Next the practitioner bends his knees, tucks his tailbone under and contracts his abdomen, trying to bring his navel to the point directly opposite on the backbone, while slowly inhaling. The mind is focused on bringing the two points together. The position is held as long as is comfortable. The exercise ends with a Half Basic and a Basic.

1.35 | WASHING THE STOMACH METHOD
Digestive System

T HIS EXERCISE works from a mechanical point of view by literally washing the Stomach with tea (Tea Bo Nay is an excellent choice), and from an energetic point of view by stimulating ST 25.

ST 25, known as Heaven's Pivot is an interesting acupoint. Both the Small Intestine and the Large Intestine are intimately related to the energy of the Stomach. It is the point on the front of the body where the energy of the Large Intestine gathers and we have seen before how important the Large Intestine is in excreting waste and fueling the Ming Men. The point is extremely effective in draining pathological dampness from the Lower Burner and eliminating stasis. ST 25 treats the widest variety of intestinal disharmonies.

The name Heaven's Pivot reflects its central position beside the navel. The area above this point is said to be ruled by Heaven's Chi and the area below by Earth's Chi. The area where these two manifestations of Chi meet is the place where man's Chi begins.

The exercise begins with the practitioner drinking a cup of tea. He then raises his hands to the level of the head while inhaling, drops his fists to the lower abdomen while swallowing energy to the Lower Tan Tien and follows with the POOH sound. Then with both hands he pinches the skin on ST 25—to the left side of the navel on the lateral border of the rectus abdominis muscle. While breathing normally, he rotates the pinched skin eighteen times clockwise, sucking in his abdomen and pushing it out once during each rotation. Concluding with a Basic he repeats the same technique on the same side but rotating the pinched skin in the opposite direction. The exercise is only done on the left side.

STRATEGY NOTE | *After energizing and clearing the area where we began as men, the last exercise activates the highest expression of our physical selves—the area where Jing holds Original Spirit embodied.*

1.36 | ENERGY FLOW TO THE TOP
Sea of Marrow

THIS EXERCISE concentrates energy in the Sea of Marrow and specifically at GV 20.

GV 20, known as Hundred Meetings, is the uppermost acupoint on the body. It is the meeting point of all the Yang energy of the body in general and specifically the place where the Governing Vessel meets the Urinary Bladder, Triple Burner, and Gall Bladder. An internal branch of the Liver Channel also rises to GV 20. Interestingly, the Jing exercises began with the Liver Organ and are ending with a point that brings the influence of the Liver to the highest point of the body. Indeed it is the highest direct extension of any Yin Organ.

GV 20 has the ability to raise Yang energy in the Governing Vessel. It is through this point that energy from Heaven is most easily assimilated.

The Sea of Marrow is generated from the essence of the Kidneys. When two essences come together Spirit arrives. By nourishing the essences of the brain, we provide the opportunity to enrich our Spiritual content.

Some traditions contend that a mixture of the Jing from the Sea of Marrow and energy from Heaven can mix and form an "Immortal Body" which can leave the physical body with full consciousness and essentially "cheat death." Most traditions agree that it is a portal to other dimensions.

Activating GV 20 will energize the Pineal Gland (body's biological clock), Thalamus (center of sensory stimuli), and Hypothalamus (control of entire hormonal system) and the Pituitary Gland (master gland of the body).

The exercise begins with the practitioner standing with feet less than shoulder width and the hands at the sides. The hands are raised to the level of the head while inhaling and dropped to the lower abdomen in fists while swallowing to the Lower Tan Tien. The POOH sound is then made.

The practitioner then raises his open palms to the level of the upper chest while slowly inhaling and concentrating energy at the top of the head—GV 20. The position is held as long as comfortable. The exercise ends with a Half Basic and a Basic.

This completes the thirty six exercises of Level 1.

STRATEGY NOTE | *The process of refinement through Chi Kung practice is cumulative. The exercises must be practiced regularly, and as time goes on their effects will become more apparent and infinitely more profound. Chan Chiu Lim spoke very little in the years I spent with him, but the two things he did repeat often were: "The Chi is Unlimited" and "Nothing real comes quickly."*

The keys to successful cultivation are: to have a complete system correctly transmitted from which to do the work, to train regularly, to train regularly, and to train regularly. In the words of Sifu Chan: "continue, continue, continue!" ☯

CHAPTER 5

Introduction to Level 2

THIS SECOND LEVEL in the *Strategies* series attempts the formidable task of intellectualizing processes in the body which are profound in theory and elusive in practice. The thirty six exercises in the Second Level can be described and their underlying theory explained, but the essential result of their practice activates a mystical union of forces that defies substantial description.

Chi, the Second Level of Hua Shan Taoist Chi Kung, is concerned with uniting the basic Yin/Yang energies of the body as represented by Fire and Water. The Chi referred to at this level is not one of the many forms of Chi that support the normal functions of life for the average human being. These energies correspond with the First Level of training, energies that build, support and maintain the physical form.

Exercises in this Second Level deal with enriching, vitalizing and harmonizing the basic Fire and Water of the body, causing them to interact in such a way that latent potentials of both body and mind are activated and the pathways which support spiritual evolvement are opened.

It is hoped that by describing the individual strategies of each of the thirty six exercises and the overall strategy of their placement in the system, the reader will begin to get a "feeling" for the alchemical processes that can be stimulated in the body.

By necessity these explanations will appear as linear three dimensional constructs. It is important to remember that human attributes are often multi-functional and as beings we are multidimensional. Processes that are explained in one time and geographic frame may be occurring simultaneously with numerous other processes dimensionally differentiated.

CHAPTER 6

Background

THE EXERCISES in Chapter 4 explaining the First Level of Han Shan Taoist Chi Kung were fairly easily understood as methods to develop and strengthen the physical form and functional energies that manifest as a human being. Explaining the Second Level necessitates a deep understanding of the energetic construction of the body and a clear conception of exactly what the exercises are trying to accomplish.

The following quote from Chapter 3 (*see pg. 35*) will set the stage for our exploration of the SECOND LEVEL | Chi (Energy);

> "To understand the pathways of Hua Shan Taoist Chi Kung, we must look at the overall energetic potentials both manifest and unmanifest of the human being."

In theory, there are four basic degrees of human consciousness or potential:

The **First Degree** is represented by Divine Spirit. It is the state of singularity beyond Yin and Yang. Reaching this state is the highest aim of spiritual disciplines.

The **Second Degree** is represented by the harmonious interaction of Yin and Yang. Both principles are present but have not yet differentiated. This is the level of the Source/Ming Men origin of the Pericardium/Triple Burner duality and wellspring of the Eight Extra-Ordinary Vessels.

The **Third Degree** is where Yin and Yang differentiate to manifest Water and Fire; their basic representatives in Man.

The **Fourth Degree** embodies the results from the activities and interactions of Water and Fire. These include the Five Elemental (Phase) Energies, the Eight Extra-Ordinary Vessels, the Twelve Regular Meridians, and all the structures, rhythms and functions of the body.

The pathway of development in Hua Shan Taoist Chi Kung leads the practitioner from the fourth Degree upward to ultimately unite with the Divine.

> LEVEL 1 | **Essence** (Jing) exercises work at the level of the Fourth Degree, supporting proper functioning of all the energies and functions at that level.

> LEVEL 2 | **Energy** (Chi) exercises work at the level of the Third Degree, supporting the transforming interactions of Yin and Yang, Water and Fire that provide more refined energies to approach higher consciousness.

> LEVEL 3 | **Spirit** (Shen) exercises which work at the level of the Second Degree, address the co-penetration of the refined energies from Level 2 with the embodied Spirit of the individual to open the doorway for reception of Divine Grace.

It should be stated here that some authorities recognize only Three Degrees of consciousness, maintaining the Divine and undifferentiated Yin and Yang (First and Second Degrees) are, in fact, the same state. This view of reality in no way interferes with the underlying philosophy of Hua Shan Taoist Chi Kung. Shen exercises bring the practitioner to the state of singularity that opens one to Divinity. One can, by his own exertions, go no further. Divine Grace, from whatever philosophical realm, manifests according to its own way. ☯

CHAPTER 7

Origins

FIRST DEGREE

THE FIRST DEGREE is the realm of the Divine. It is beyond Yin and Yang, beyond the possibility of conception by the human intellect.

SECOND DEGREE

HUMAN BEINGS are a mixture of what are referred to as "Prenatal and Postnatal energies."

Prenatal energies are our constitutional heritage derived from both our parents and the Divine. They are the foundation of our general physical and energetic make-up. The ancient Chinese classics say that when two Essences come together the Spirit arrives and that when two Spirits come together form is initiated.

Before conception, the Essences (Jing) of the mother and the father come together attracting Divine Spirit (Shen). The co-penetration of these Prenatal Essences and Shen express Prenatal Chi. These three prenatal potentials (Original Jing, Shen, and Chi) are fused as the singularity preceding our development as human beings. Without material manifestation, they form an interfunctional unit that directs our course from preconception to post materialization. The place where these Three Original Treasures co-penetrate is called the Ming Men or 'Gate of Life.'

Ming Men is the first and most important energy center in the body. First because it is formed at the moment of conception, even before the fetus is formed and, most important because it is the center of energetic transformations.

Bilateral Ming Men, located in the Kidneys, has seven energy channels connecting its two sides called the "Moving Chi between the Kidneys." This is where Heaven and Earth meet in Man and interact to produce life. Prenatal Chi, Postnatal Chi, and Cosmic Energy interface and transform in Ming Men to support life. It is the origin of the Governing Vessel, the Conception Vessel, Chong Mai, and the Triple Burner.

"Ming Men is often considered the back of the Lower Tan Tien. In fact, the Lower Tan Tien, Moving Chi between the Kidneys and Ming Men are so intimately connected that they can be considered one."—*see Chapter 1, pg. 14*

Postnatal energies are generated from the environment after birth. The body utilizes breath from Heaven via the Lungs and food and water from Earth via the digestive system to supplement the original energies to support our lives. Postnatal Jing is formed from the result of metabolized food and water from Earth, Postnatal Shen is formed from inhaling 'the breaths of Heaven,' and Postnatal Chi results from metabolism of both the breath and food and water.

THIRD DEGREE

IN ANCIENT CHINESE classics, the first manifestation coming from the One was Light. The Light condensed to Water. The ancient symbol for Water is the trigram:

▬▬▬▬ ▬▬▬▬	Yin line
▬▬▬▬▬▬▬▬▬▬	Yang line
▬▬▬▬ ▬▬▬▬	Yin line

Water is a Yin substance, yet its innermost part is considered Yang. Yang relates to Fire. It is from the innermost part of Water that the Yang of Fire differentiated itself and produced Earth. Earth then generated the '10,000 things.'

The level of the Third Degree represents the differentiation of the One into basic Fire and Water from which spring the 10,000 things. This level encompasses the relationships of all the polar opposites that mutually support the grosser energies of the Fourth Degree.

These polar opposites express themselves in the Fourth Degree through three energy systems. The Ming Men proper extends itself in two channels on each side of the spine. The Governing Vessel and Conception Vessel represent the primal polarities in the Extra-Ordinary Meridian System, and the Triple Burner and Pericardium represent the polarities that precurse the energies of the five Elements. These three systems will be explored in the next chapter.

In Taoist Chi Kung, working at the level of the Third Degree is said to "bring youthfulness back from old age." The latent energies activated by exercises that affect this level are closer to the Source, of a much higher potency and vibration, and capable of exerting enormous influence on the lower vibrational energetics of the Fourth Degree while opening the pathways to the Divine.

FOURTH DEGREE

THE FOURTH DEGREE encompasses all the energies structured by the Eight Extra-Ordinary Vessels and manifested as extensions of the Five Elemental Phases.

"The Eight Extra-Ordinary Meridians are vital aspects of our most primitive constitution. They are the initial organizers of those forces that will produce our being and remain fundamental distributors of Essence, Chi and Spirit throughout our lives. They represent the organizational parameters of the body, controlling the powers that create and balance our personal manifestation of the union of energies that precede our form. The Eight Extra-Ordinary Meridians organize the original Yin and Yang of our bodies.

The Eight Extra-Ordinary Meridians are often viewed as reservoirs of energy for the rest of the body, accepting excess energy from the system and releasing energy to deficient areas. They preserve normal functioning of the body at the deepest levels.

The Governing Vessel expresses Chi and Yang at the deepest level. The Conception Vessel expresses Blood and Yin. The Chong Mai is the bursting forth of life from the original Yin and Yang while the Dai Mai provides boundaries for that life. Yin and Yang Chiao Mai regulate the rhythms and interpenetration of Yin and Yang, while Yin and Yang Wei Mai organize the systems of Blood and Yin and Chi and Yang. From these original organizations spring the functional responsibilities of the Twelve Regular Meridians and their Organs." —*Strategies Taoist Chi Kung, Chapter 1 (see pg. 14 & 15)*

Although the Triple Burner and Pericardium are depicted as constituents of the Fire Elements on most Five Element charts, many scholars contend that they retain attributes of both Fire and Water and are intermediary between the Source and the functional Five Elements.

The Pericardium masters all the vital circulation relating to Blood in the body and the Triple Burner controls the diversity and unity of Chi in the body.

The Five Elements are Wood, Fire, Earth, Metal and Water. These terms do not denote the actual physical manifestations of wood, fire, earth, metal and water. They represent energetic qualities associated with these manifestations.

The ancients observed the natural cycles of birth, growth, maturity, harvest, and storage. The energetic properties of these cycles or phases were the framework upon which the theory of the Five Elements was constructed.

Five Element energetic actions and interactions are involved in the constantly changing play of life in regular observable cycles. Every aspect of the universe can be associated with some aspect of the Five Element Theory.

Man is said to be the manifestation of the very best of the Five Element Energies. As with the universe at large, every aspect of man, including the mind, emotions and physical substances can be explained by and associated with Five Element Correspondences. ☯

Five Element Correspondences

	Wood	*Fire*	*Earth*	*Metal*	*Water*
Viscera	liver	heart	spleen	lung	kidney
Bowel	gall bladder	small intestine	stomach	large intestine	urinary bladder
Color	green	red	yellow	white	black/blue
Emotion	anger	joy	reminis-cence	grief/sorrow	fear/fright
Tissue	tendon	blood vessels	muscle	skin/sense	bone
Sense Organ	eyes	tongue	mouth	nose	ears
Season	sping	summer	late summer	fall	winter
Taste	sour	bitter	sweet	pungent	salty
Direction	east	south	middle	west	north
Climate	wind	heat	damp	dry	cold
Nature	birth	growth	mature	harvest	store
Sound	shout	laugh	sing	weep	groan
Liquid Emitted	tears	sweat	saliva	mucous	urine
Grain	wheat	millet	rye	rice	beans
Meat	chicken	mutton	beef	horse	pork
Nourishes	nails	complexion	lips	body hair	head hair

CHAPTER 8

Level 2 | Energy (Chi)

AS STATED BEFORE, the Chi referred to at this level is not one of the regular functional aspects of Chi that is involved with the normal workings of the body. The Chi activated at this level is the latent potential inherent in all human beings which results from the harmonization of the basic polarity underlying our existence as individuals. This power is in effect downgraded to facilitate our manifestation as embodied beings.

Exercises in the Second Level of Hua Shan Taoist Chi Kung are designed to support the harmonization of the two polar opposites, producing a highly refined Chi. This powerful, refined Chi, being the link between man and singularity, can access both our Original Three Treasure Complex and the specialized energetic systems that comprise our life as individuals.

Activating this Chi has always been a risky business. If the lower vibrational energy systems (including body/mind/emotion aspects) that comprise our life are not in balance themselves or are unprepared for the exponential power surge of Chi, problems can result. Writings from the ancients and direct lineage teachers from the present constantly warn practitioners not to enter these areas of study without the guidance of an experienced teacher.

Safety is one of the main reasons why many ancient systems have been held as "secret." The proper preparation for access to these higher energies by practitioners is a long process. The process entails years of practice, balancing and strengthening the body-mind complex to not only access this higher vibrational energy but to actually benefit from its presence.

There are many instances of students prematurely accessing these energies and experiencing detrimental effects to both body and mind. The old texts warn that the results of embarking on the "short path" are sickness, insanity, death, or enlightenment. One chance in four of a positive result comes from "having a sincere student follow a complete system with a good guide."

As more and more people are interested in studying ancient systems of energetic development, the danger of well meaning practitioners wanting to share the wonder of the journey with others increases. Students and teachers alike should be careful that the information shared is complete and presented in the correct order. There is an appropriate timing for the presentation of techniques in any system. Advanced practices will at best be useless to unprepared students and at worst may be harmful.

With the increasing access to energetic systems available in modern times, another danger is the mixing and matching of systems —'chop suey kung fooy.' In the past, students were lucky to have one system available to them and tended to spend long periods of time learning the teachings of one lineage. With a firm background in one system, they were able to study and evaluate other practices more wisely.

In modern times, it is common for students to jump from one system to another, often spending only a few years in each. This leaves them with an incomplete understanding of the "big picture" and the possibility of either missing important pieces of the puzzle, thereby never progressing beyond the beginning stages or becoming unbalanced through incomplete or untimely practice.

THEORY

WE WILL EXPLORE the Level 2 | Chi theory by taking a look at five pairs of "opposites" that the thirty six exercises in this level either directly access and harmonize or indirectly support. Those "opposites" are the Yin/Yang aspects of the Ming Men, the basic Fire (Middle Tan Tien) and Water (Lower Tan Tien) of the body, and the Governing and Conception Vessels.

The Lower Tan Tien/Ming Men internal connection and the Lower Tan Tien/Ming Men external connection, although technically not paired opposites, are important pathways for linking Yin and Yang in the body.

The Yin/Yang aspects of the Ming Men as specific channels are not often discussed in Taoist Literature. In Esoteric Buddhism and Yoga they are called the 'Two Side Channels' (Ida and Pingala) and occupy an important position in the theory of Yoga practices.

On the other hand, the Governing and Conception Vessels are little discussed in Yoga and Esoteric Buddhism but play a major role in the theory of Taoist Practices.

The basic Fire and Water of the body are utilized by practitioners of all three lineages. For Yoga practitioners and Esoteric Buddhists, they relate to Prana and Apana, while for Taoists they relate to the Middle Tan Tien and the Lower Tan Tien.

The internal connection of the Lower Tan Tien/Ming Men relates to the Uddiyana Bandha or 'abdominal lock' in Yoga and various abdominal muscle contracting breathing techniques in Taoist Practices.

The external connection of the Lower Tan Tien/Ming Men is associated with activity in the Dai Mai or 'Belt Channel' and is seldom discussed in any literature.

All five pairs of "opposites" are directly connected to the Ming Men/Source and, despite cultural dispositions to intellectually accent one or the other, in practice all five are utilized by each system to initiate access to higher vibrational energies. The ultimate goal of each harmonization is to generate refined Chi that will open the Central Channel (Chong Mai) and energize the highest centers in the body to ultimately merge with Universal Presence.

THE TWO SIDE CHANNELS

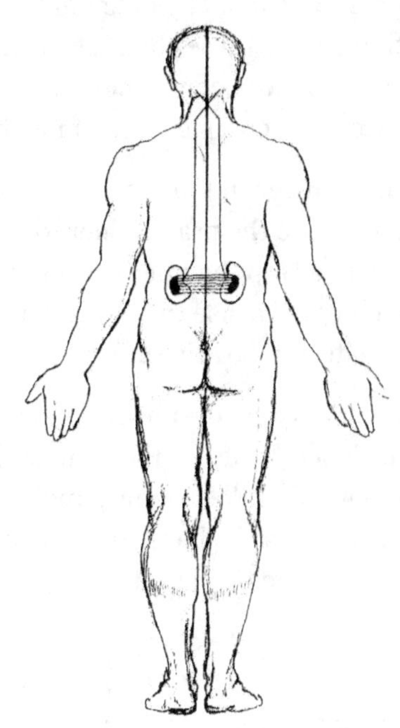

Ming Men

THE TWO SIDE CHANNELS are direct extensions of the Ming Men, repository of the Original Yin and Yang of the body/mind/spirit complex. They are little mentioned in Taoist lineages. Hua Shan Taoist Chi Kung uses these channels extensively. In Yoga texts, the channels are named Ida and Pingala and are also sometimes called the Sun and Moon channels. Sun and Moon are names used for these channels in Hua Shan Chi Kung. These terms, Sun and Moon, are used in Taoist references to describe the basic Yin/Yang energies in the Tan Tien. Ida refers to the Left Side Channel. It is said to relate to the Yin qualities of water, feminine, night, negative, cold, moon, mental activity, intuition, desire, subconscious mind, passive, internal, parasympathetic nervous system, etc.

Pingala refers to the Right Side Channel. It is said to relate to the Yang qualities of fire, masculine, daytime, positive, hot, sun, physical activity, logic, action, conscious mind, active, external, sympathetic nervous system, etc.

Ida and Pingala are believed to function alternately. The goal of Chi exercises is to increase the vitality in each channel and to harmonize their activities. This vitalization and harmonization activates the powerful latent energies of the body and opens the Central Channel—the Sushumna or Chong Mai. Spiritual evolution is the result of these forces combining and rising through the Central Channel to the brain (thus nourishing the Spirit).

Because this level of training involves such powerful potentials, great care must be taken in teaching and practicing techniques that access these channels. Improper activation of these energies can have dire consequences. A careful, well-monitored approach through a complete system is the only safe pathway to progress.

Imbalances in Ida are said to produce wild psychic experiences and cause the practitioner to become withdrawn. Imbalances in Pingala trap the practitioner in worldly experiences. Either extreme will cause the practitioner to deplete his vital energies and negate any positive effects derived from his training.

The thirty six exercises in the Level 1—Essence (Jing) category are designed to purify the form and functions of the body, harmonize the mind and emotions, and strengthen the nervous system to provide a safe "base" from which the practitioner can begin to work at the Chi Level.

The thirty six exercises in the Level 2—Energy (Chi) category are designed to safely energize and harmonize our basic polarities in order to facilitate progress to the level of nourishing the Spirit.

THE GOVERNING VESSEL
AND CONCEPTION VESSEL

THE GOVERNING VESSEL (Yang) and the Conception Vessel (Yin) are pathways that are usually accessed by Taoist practitioners for working at the Chi Level. Both Vessels originate in the Ming Men/Tan Tien and are often referred to as the Yin and Yang of the Source.

The Governing Vessel is called the 'Sea of Yang' because it regulates all the Yang of the body. It's external channel begins in the perineum, follows the midline of the back to the head, and ends just below the nose.

The Conception Vessel is responsible for all the Yin of the body. It's external channel begins in the perineum, follows the midline up the front of the body and ends just below the mouth.

These two Vessels are considered to be of primary importance by Taoist Chi Kung practitioners for precisely the reasons described above; they control the Yin and Yang of the whole body.
Some authorities state that the Governing Vessel is associated with Chi and Water (Kidneys), the Conception Vessel is associated with Blood and Fire (Heart), and that all form and functions of the body depend on them.

It follows that the Governing Vessel and Conception Vessel, when properly linked and energized, can harmonize all the Yin and Yang and Fire and Water aspects of the body—precisely the goal of Chi exercises.

We will explore both these channels in more detail as the exercises that are specific to each are described.

FIRE AND WATER

FOR TAOISTS working with Fire and Water, it means working with energies of the Lower Tan Tien and the Middle Tan Tien, while for Yoga practitioners, it means working with Apana and Prana.

The Lower Tan lien is located just below the navel. Authorities differ on its exact location and, in fact, the location can vary in different individuals. The perception of the location of the Lower Tan Tien can change for each individual at various stages of training. Complete Chi Kung systems will provide the tools for the student's relationship with the Lower Tan Tien to become closer and more exact as his practice matures.

The Lower Tan Tien is the foundation of the body and the root of all Taoist Practices. It is the original source of energy, both as the original area of conception and the area where sustenance enters the body from the mother via the umbilical cord. It not only stores the Original Chi/Prenatal Chi (derived from parents at conception), but also acts as a storehouse where Chi from all sources is collected, blended and transformed.

The Lower Tan Tien is the underlying energetic substratum around which revolve all other energetic manifestations in the body, and is a manifestation of an even more profound universal energy. It is here that the energy of Heaven, Earth and Man interface.

The energies of the Lower Tan Tien are considered to represent Water because of their close association with the Kidney and the Source.

The Middle Tan Tien is located in the center of the chest at CV 17, directly between the nipples in men. The area is called the Sea of Chi, because it is the meeting point of all the Chi of the body. It is also the front gathering point of the Pericardium which will be discussed shortly.

The Chi that is produced from the environment through the digestive process and breathing is gathered in the 'Sea of Chi.' This Chi is the result of a burning process and so is related to Fire. The 'Sea of Chi' or Middle Tan Tien is also intimately related to the Heart and Pericardium (Fire Element). This deepens its relationship with Fire.

In Chi Level exercises, the prenatal energy from the Lower Tan Tien (Water) is mixed with the postnatal energy from the Middle Tan Tien (Fire) to refine more intense energies that will activate later potentials for spiritual growth.

No discussion of the Chi Level would be complete without exploring the roles of the Pericardium and Triple Burner; functions which are related to both Fire and Water.

PERICARDIUM AND TRIPLE BURNER

THE PERICARDIUM and Triple Burner are, in fact, the dominant force potentials inherent at this level. Both are intimately related to the Source, acting as extensions of the basic polarities that precede all material and energetic manifestations. They are the first emissaries of Yin and Yang symbolizing Fire and Water in the body. The Pericardium and Triple Burner are like transformers that moderate the intensities of our primal energies so that we may embody. This, of course, is why we work at this level to access that "from which we embodied."

The Pericardium, as the vehicle through which the 'Sovereign Heart' communicates with the rest of the body, is directly related to (in some texts synonymous with) the Middle Tan Tien or 'Sea of Chi.' The Pericardium is the functional aspect of the Heart, controlling Blood and the network of channels that deliver Blood throughout the body. It is through the Spirits infused in the Blood by the Heart that we fulfill our destiny and through the nutrients or essences carried by the Blood that we nourish our body/mind/spirit complex.

The Triple Burner is said to be the 'pathway of water and grain' or the beginning and end of Chi. The Triple Burner is the messenger of the Source, bringing Source Chi to all the meridians. Both prenatal Chi and postnatal Chi are dependent on the Triple Burner to function in the body.

"The Triple Burner is a generalization of the functions of the organs in three areas of the body. The Upper Burner represents the chest and functions of the Heart and Lungs in transporting Blood and Chi. The Middle Burner represents the epigastrium and the functions of the Spleen/Stomach in digestion and absorption. The Lower Burner represents the hypogastrium and functions of the Kidney/Urinary Bladder and Large Intestine in controlling water metabolism and the excretion of waste products. The Triple Burner belongs to the Fire Element and is related to the South." —*see Horse Riding 2, exercise 1.8, pg. 49*

Beyond the obvious functional responsibilities outlined above, the Triple Burner plays a germane role in all activities of the body. Ming Men is the 'original energy of life,' and Yin (Water) and Yang (Fire) are the first differentiation of that energy in the living being. The Triple Burner is the vehicle through which the interactions of that first differentiation build and support life. It links whatever follows to the Source and extends the power of the Source throughout the body. The Triple Burner transports Jing, Chi and Shen throughout the body.

The Pericardium and Triple Burner are responsible for all the Fire/Water interactions in the body. In many ways, the merging of Lower Tan Tien energy and Middle Tan Tien energy is precisely reversing the "transformer effect" and making high intensity energy available to both rejuvenate the body and accelerate spiritual evolvement.

From the Yoga point of view, there are five Vayus similar to the Five Element concept of the Chinese Systems. Each Vayu has an energetic function and an area of operation in the body.

The function associated with Prana Vayu, located in the area of the Middle Tan Tien, is absorption of Prana from the environment. Prana Vayu is directly related to Ida or the Left Side Channel.

The process of elimination through the genito/urinary and excretory systems is controlled by Apana Vayu, located in the area of the Lower Tan Tien. This Vayu is directly related to Pingala or the Right Side Channel.

Apana has a tendency to flow downwards and Prana flows upwards. These normal outward flowing tendencies result in loss of energy. The Yogic texts state that if you can reverse the downward flow of Apana and the upward flow of Prana, causing them to flow inward, reversal of the aging process is possible. For Taoists, this corresponds to the mixing of energies from the Lower Tan Tien and the Middle Tan Tien. The Yoga theory clearly relates these two areas to the Two Side Channels.

In summary, work at the Chi Level is all about bringing together the various manifestations of Original Yin and Yang, Fire and Water. This communication of energies initiates the potentials for more powerful energies to open the pathways of spiritual evolution on the one hand and to rejuvenate our body/mind/spirit complex on the other.

INTERNAL CONNECTION OF THE LOWER
TAN TIEN/MING MEN

THIS INTERNAL CONNECTION of Yin and Yang is made by mechanically bringing the front and back of the abdomen together. By directing the energies of the Ming Men point on the backbone and the Lower Tan Tien area of the abdomen to move toward each other, a joining of the basic Source Polarities is accomplished. This meeting, as with the other four meetings, produces heat, which initiates opening of the Central Channel and subsequent nourishment of the Spirit. 'Heating the Life Door' (see exercise 1.34, pg.83) is a perfect example of this technique.

EXTERNAL CONNECTION OF THE LOWER
TAN TIEN/MING MEN

THIS EXTERNAL CONNECTION is accomplished through activating the Belt Channel. The Belt Channel circles the Lower Tan Tien/Ming Men area. Energy flowing through this channel mixes and balances the basic Source Polarities. One way of activating the Belt Channel is by energizing the Gall Bladder Meridian. This technique is used throughout the system, especially by turning the head from side to side. ☯

CHAPTER 9

Exercises for Level 2 | Chi

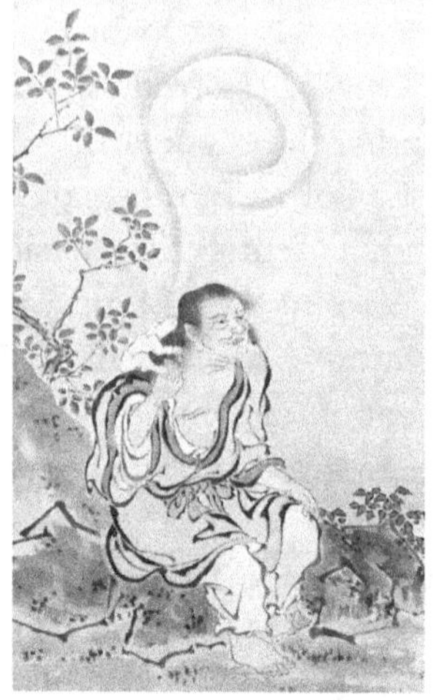

B Y T H E T I M E the student begins work on these exercises, he has been well grounded in the thirty six exercises of the Essence Level. This does not mean that the Essence Level exercises have been perfected, only that enough time has been spent doing them to make the next level safe for training.

Although the exercises in each level are energetically different, they do not exist in a vacuum. The practitioner's development mediates the effects of the exercises. Each Level is designed both to support increased energetic development in the practitioner and to provide a broad base from which he may safely progress to higher Levels.

As this is a book on the underlying strategies of the system and not an instruction manual, the descriptions of the exercises are meant to show how they effect development and why they occupy their place in the system. The descriptions should not be taken as instructions. (They are meant for information and educational purposes only!)

This book will have served its purpose if it provides sufficient food for thought to help practitioners of many lineages understand their own systems more fully.

Most exercises in this Level begin with raising the open hands to the level of the head while inhaling, swallowing energy to the Lower Tan Tien while dropping the hands (in fists) to the lower abdomen and making the POOH sound. This beginning, which was often seen in Level 1, takes on more significance at Level 2 because it initiates the process of mixing Fire and Water, Yin and Yang.

Energy in the body has a tendency to follow the related movement of the hands. Bringing the hands up leads the energy up and bringing the hands down leads the energy down. The up and down motions both aid the Lower and Upper Tan Tiens in communicating and increase circulation in the Governing Vessel and Conception Vessel. The forming of fists as the hands reach the lower abdomen helps 'fix' energy in the Lower Tan Tien. To save space, this beginning technique will simply be called Gathering Energy in the Lower Tan Tien.

LEVEL 2 | EXERCISES FOR CHI

2.1 | MOVING THE ENERGY UP AND DOWN TO TWO SIDES

THIS EXERCISE is somewhat of a combination of Moving the Energy Up and Down and Centering the Energy, both from Level 1. Although similar in form to the Level 1 exercises, the functions corresponding to those forms are different.

After Gathering the Energy in the Lower Tan Tien, the first movement of Moving the Energy Up and Down to Two Sides is identical to the first movement of Moving the Energy Up and Down in Level 1 which is then followed by a swallow of energy to the Lower Tan Tien and a POOH. This is the only exercise in the system that performs two swallows and POOHS in a row.

In this case the purpose of the movement is not to begin the process of moving energy in the body but rather to center the energy in the Lower Tan Tien (and collect energy via the swallow). The left side of the body is considered Yang and the right side is Yin. Yin energy tends to move downward and Yang energy moves upward. By raising the right arm and lowering the left arm, the natural movements of these energies are brought to neutral. The swallow consolidates the energy in the Lower Tan Tien, as does the subsequent return of the fists to the lower abdomen.

The exercise continues with the practitioner bending forward at 90°, turning to the left and exhaling while extending his arms downward and out to the sides up to shoulder level.

In Centering the Energy *(see Centering the Energy, exercise 1.9, pg. 50)*, exhaling in this bent over position is used to direct energy to the Lower Tan Tien, encouraged by the placement of the hands at the waist.

In the present exercise, the same exhale and body position, with the exception of the arms, is used to direct energy from the Lower Tan Tien to the Middle Tan Tien. The different effect results from the arm movement directing the energy upwards while simultaneously opening and expanding the chest.

The practitioner then straightens his waist while inhaling, swallows to the Lower Tan Tien and brings his fists back to the lower abdomen. This gathers energy into the Lower Tan Tien again. He then bends his waist at 90° and turns to the right side, repeating the exercise on that side. The exercise ends with a Half Basic and a Basic.

In this exercise, the breath and body positions increase communication between the Lower and Middle Tan Tiens. The same conditions initiate circulation in the Governing Vessel *(see Yang Pulse, exercise 2.10, pg. 120)*, Conception Vessel *(see Yin Pulse, exercise 2.9, pg. 119)* and Chong Mai *(see Energy to Chong Mai, exercise 2.5, pg. 112)*. The turning from side to side activates the Two

Side Channels and the bending stimulates Ming Men.

In terms of Level 2 energetic pathways, this exercise utilizes all three. Because it ends with the energy in the Middle Tan Tien, the overall effect is to slightly favor the raising of energy from the Lower Tan Tien to the Middle Tan Tien—Jing to Chi—as the formula goes.

2.2 | ENERGY TO FINGERS

THIS IS A SIMPLE yet powerful exercise. After Gathering Energy in the Lower Tan Tien, the hands are held in open "claws" and rotated in extended circles between the Lower Tan Tien and Middle Tan Tien while performing a long, slow inhale. The exercise ends with a Basic.

The pathways of the circles bring the hands close to the body on the upward cycle and have them descend away from the body. This pattern biases the communication in the Jing to Chi direction as the energy inside the body follows the hand movements.

The formation of the hands, with the palms spread, activates the Pericardium through P 8, one of the most important acupoints used in Taoist Chi Kung. P 8, known as 'Palace of Toil,' is the major point on the upper limbs that allows the energy of the body to communicate with the external world. It is also the major point for emitting Chi from the body for healing purposes. Development of P 8 allows energy to flow from the body out to the universe and allows universal energy to be absorbed into the body.

TB 4 is the Source point of the Triple Burner, the point where Source Energy directly communicates with the Triple Burner Meridian. TB 4 is located on the back of the hands and has a special relationship with energy in all of the fingers, so by concentrating energy in the fingers the Triple Burner is activated through TB 4.

The movement of the back during the exercise stimulates the Two Side Channels (each side alternately expanding and compressing). The long slow inhale stimulates the Lower Tan Tien/Ming Men Complex.

The revolving of the hands and the internal movement it causes also stimulates the Governing and Conception Vessels. This is
facilitated by the bowed spine position assumed in the exercise and
by placing the tongue on the roof of the mouth to connect
the two vessels.

Again, this exercise uses all three energetic pathways focused on in
Level 2 and biases the movement of energy from Jing to Chi.

2.3 | ENERGY TO THE UPPER ARMS, BACK OF NECK & HEAD

THIS EXERCISE is extremely intense and is **contra-indicat-
ed for anyone with high blood pressure.** It drastically
increases the amount of blood and energy flowing to the brain and
is therefore thought to increase intelligence.

After Gathering Energy in the Lower Tan Tien, the arms are locked
in a particular fashion and another breath is inhaled. Then the
practitioner bends forward forcing the energy in the Lower Tan
Tien and Middle Tan Tien together and directing blood and energy
to the head.

The joining of the energy in the Two Tan Tiens is the precursor to
refined energy rising up to nourish the Spirit. This exercise accomplishes the joining and the rising mechanically. It is a gross way
of opening the pathways that will be used for transporting more
refined energies when the practitioner is more developed.

STRATEGY NOTE | *The first three exercises in Level 2 have
utilized various techniques to bring the opposing polarities of the
body together and to encourage energy to rise from the Lower
Tan Tien upward bringing Jing to Chi. This upward rising energy
can be problematical if it is not balanced by appropriate downward energy. The uprising energy is classified as Yang/hot and
must be balanced by downward moving Yin/cool energy. The
negative result of unbalanced energy rising is called "Kundalini
Syndrome" in the Yoga community and "burning the heart and/or*

burning the brain" in Chi Kung circles. A wide array of symptoms can result from this disharmony, from simple problems to life-threatening conditions. Proper functioning of the Governing Vessel/Conception Vessel circuit (see Little Earth, exercise 2.11, Pg. 121) is the main safety valve for preventing this condition in Taoist Chi Kung. Little Earth not only offers safety from imbalances, but also recycles extra energies for rejuvenating the body. Making sure all the energetic pathways to the feet are open and free flowing is another safety technique utilized in Hua Shan Taoist Chi Kung.

2.4 | SALIVA TO TAN TIEN

SALIVA TO THE TAN TIEN is an exercise common to many styles of Chi Kung. Our version entails Gathering Energy in the Lower Tan Tien, followed by clicking the teeth together thirty six times. The saliva generated is then swallowed to the Lower Tan Tien and the exercise is completed with a Basic. The whole process is repeated four more times. Swallowing saliva is a powerful aid to opening the Conception Vessel (protection) and a technique for nourishing the internal organs.

It is generally acknowledged that clicking the teeth together moves energy in the bones and marrow (via the Kidney/bones/marrow connection) and strengthens the connection between the Governing and Conception Vessels—similar to putting the tongue on the roof of the mouth.

In Chi Kung practice, the saliva generated is always swallowed. Taoists consider saliva itself a valuable substance. The Two Side Channels cross at the back of the head and branch to the root of the tongue. Saliva is thought to be derived from the Essence of Ming Men and is capable of improving digestive function, generating Blood in the Heart, improving eyesight through Liver supplementation, promoting body fluids via the Spleen, strengthening Lung Chi, and nourishing the Kidney Essence.

The saliva produced by Chi Kung practice is thought to be

especially valuable due to the active state of the Ming Men at that time. Another time when the Ming Men is active is during sexual activity. The saliva produced by both sexual activity and Chi Kung practice usually has a sweeter taste than ordinary saliva and is much more potent. Trading saliva with a sexual partner is practiced by some as a means of energetic cultivation.

STRATEGY NOTE | *Practicing Saliva to the Tan Tien at this point in the system gathers the fruit of the upward moving energy generated in the first three exercises and brings it to the Lower Tan Tien, both as a safety procedure and as additional nourishment for the overall being.*

2.5 | ENERGY TO CHONG MAI

CHONG MAI is the Central Channel—the main pathway to nourish the Spirit with refined energy. It has always been associated with a route of communication and vigorous animation. Often called the Thrusting Channel, Chong Mai represents the Power of the Source ensuring the correct and speedy circulation of both Chi and Blood. Reflecting this dual regulation, Chong Mai is called both the Sea of Blood and the Sea of the Meridians.

Chong Mai has always been an important consideration for both Chi Kung and Yoga practitioners. In Yoga theory, it is the pathway of Sushumna to the brain. In Chi Kung theory, Chong Mai ascends through the marrow of the spinal cord to nourish the Spirit, passes through the perineum where the Yin (Conception Vessel) and Yang (Governing Vessel) meet and transform and passes through the area of the abdomen where Fire and Water meet.

Traditionally, Chong Mai originates in the lower abdomen (Ming Men/Moving Chi Between the Kidneys) along with the Governing Vessel and Conception Vessel. It descends to the perineum where one branch ascends to the brain through the spinal cord and another branch moves up to the area lateral to the midline level with the superior border of the pubic symphysis. From this point, the channel branches again. One branch joins with the Kidney Channel to eventually disperse through the chest (Sea of Chi) from which another branch ascends the throat, curves around the lips and ends under the eye. The other branch descends the medial aspect of the leg to the foot where one branch reaches the big toe, and another terminates on the sole of the foot. The branch on the sole of the foot is one reason why so many exercises in this system, especially in Levels 1 and 3, emphasize the soles of the feet. The importance of the full activation of Chong Mai cannot be underestimated.

Both the Lower Tan Tien and the chest are referred to as the 'Sea of Chi.' Chong Mai is the pathway of communication between them linking Original Chi to Acquired Chi.

The upper trajectories of Chong Mai reach the areas of both the nose and mouth. The mouth is the orifice of Earth—where the Essences of food and water enter—and the nose is the orifice where the 'Chi of Heaven' enters.

The lower trajectories access both the Yin Meridians of the foot and, through the Stomach Meridian and connecting meridians, the Yang Energy in the lower body. Chong Mai brings warmth and circulation to the Yin area of the lower body and enriches the Yang areas with essences. We know that the Governing Vessel controls the Yang of the body and that the Conception Vessel controls the Yin. Chong Mai interpenetrates and unifies the two.

Chong Mai is an interconnection between Heaven and Earth, Blood and Chi, Yin (Conception Vessel) and Yang (Governing Vessel), Fire and Water, prenatal (Kidneys) and postnatal (Stomach). Chong Mai is represented everywhere in our body/mind/spirit complex, a summation of the unity of life.

Having reviewed Chong Mai in the large sense, the purpose of Energy to Chong Mai is modest. Three important acupoints are stimulated in this exercise—TB 4, KI 13, and CV 4. TB 4 (located on the back of the wrist-bilateral) is the source point of the Triple Burner. The Triple Burner distributes Source Chi from the Kidney/Ming Men complex to the Twelve Primary Meridians, each of which has a source point to receive energy from and to communicate with the Source via the Triple Burner. TB 4 is particularly used in the Japanese Acupuncture traditions, typically with a gold needle, to strengthen Source Chi.

KI 13 (located 0. 5 body inches lateral to CV 4 bilateral) is a meeting point between the Kidney Channel and the Chong Mai. It can regulate the Conception Vessel, Chong Mai, and the Lower Burner in general.

CV 4 (located 2 body inches above the pubic symphysis on the midline of the abdomen) is the meeting point of the Conception Vessel with the Spleen, Liver and Kidney channels. This point strengthens Essence and Original Chi, regulates the Small Intestines, Lower Burner, and Urinary Bladder, tonifies the Spleen and Kidneys, benefits the uterus and restores collapse. CV 4 is often considered the lower border of the Lower Tan Tien and is one of the most important points for strengthening the body.

Whereas it is easy to see a connection between Chong Mai and these three points, none of the three is usually associated with activating Chong Mai. In fact, activation of Chong Mai directly is more a function of Level 3. An interesting fact about these three points is that all three can be used to treat abnormalities in the flow of energy in Chong Mai. Because it has such far-reaching effects and is present everywhere in the body, total activation of Chong Mai would cause the body to be one big acupoint, an energetic whole.

It should be noted that some Chi Kung practitioners recognize another branch of Chong Mai running up the center of the inside of the body. When activated, this branch is the pathway by which refined energy reaches the brain. Co-incidentally, when activated this branch expands to the spine, encompassing and merging with the branch that runs up the inside of the spine.

Energy to Chong Mai is used to strengthen the body and connect the Lower Tan Tien/Ming Men internally but, just as importantly, it is used to assure that the activity of the exercises in this Level do not produce unwanted side effects (Kundalini Syndrome, etc).

After collecting Energy in the Lower Tan Tien, this exercise uses the fingers with hands back to back (to stimulate TB 4), coupled with deep reverse breathing, to stimulate the other three points. The reverse breathing mixes the energy of the Middle Tan Tien with the energy of the Lower Tan Tien. It is interesting to note that the last movement in this exercise is an expansion of the Lower Tan Tien with an exhale. Of course, this biases the exercise towards a descension of the Middle Tan Tien energy towards the Lower Tan Tien. The exercise ends with a Basic.

2.6 | INSIDE BREATHING

INSIDE BREATHING is another very powerful technique to bring the energies of the Middle Tan Tien and the Lower Tan Tien together.

The previous exercise used the externalization of energy through reverse breathing and the pumping action of the lower abdomen to join Fire and Water. Inside Breathing uses the pumping action of the lower abdomen with no externalization of energy. It also utilizes alternating contraction and extension of the hands to magnify the effect of the "inside breathing."

After Gathering Energy in the Lower Tan Tien, the practitioner bends forward to facilitate energy flow from the Middle Tan Tien downwards. He then performs the proper number of "internal breaths" coupled with correct contraction and extension of the hands. The back to back position of the hands activates TB 4.

TB 4 (located on the back of the wrist) is the Source Point of the Triple Burner. The Triple Burner distributes Source Chi from the Kidney/Ming Men complex to the Twelve Primary Meridians, each of which has a Source Point to receive energy from and to communicate with the Source via the Triple Burner.

2.7 | ENERGY TO THE GENITALS

THIS EXERCISE is a "packing" exercise—one that utilizes continuous inhales directed to an area without exhaling. The whole genital area is engorged with energy through the practice of Energy to the Genitals. Energy is particularly focused on the external genitalia and CV 1.

After Gathering Energy in the Lower Tan Tien, six breaths are packed into the genitals. The exercise ends with a Half Basic and a Basic.

In the practice of Yoga, activation of the Vajra Nadi (channel) is said to transport physical bliss from the genitals to the head and initiate spiritual awakening in the Crown Chakra via the Sushumna Channel. Vajra Nadi originates in the area of the urethra in men and the clitoris in women, thus Vajra Nadi corresponds with one of the branches of the Governing Vessel from a Taoist point of view.

CV 1 is located in the perineum halfway between the anus and the scrotum in men or the posterior labial commmissure in women. It is known as the 'Gate of Life and Death,' 'Chi Bridge,' and the 'Meeting of Yin.'

The Gate of Life and Death refers to its regulation of sexual energy, its part in the movement of Yang energy up the spine and its ability to collect Earth energy directly from Earth energy that is channeled upwards from the legs.

CV 1 is also instrumental in preventing sexual energy from "leaking" out the lower body. Sexual energy can be transformed for enhancing health and supporting spiritual evolution by circulating it through the Conception and Governing Vessels. In fact, it is the most potent reservoir of "refinable energy" in the body.

Maintaining an abundant supply of sexual energy is a primary concern for cultivators of all traditions. The vitality of the sexual energy directly mirrors the condition of many hormones that influence aging. Sexual energy is our generative and creative force, the most powerful energy in the body.

'Chi Bridge' refers to the linking function this point has between
the Conception Vessel, Chong Mai and the Governing Vessel. It
is through this link that CV 1 supports the rising of the energy in
Chong Mai and the Governing Vessel. All Taoist Chi Kung practices
involving connecting the Conception and Governing vessels place
great emphasis on energizing CV 1.

Governing Vessel 20 is the highest point on the body and the
place where Yang gathers. Situated directly beneath GV 20 is CV 1
('Meeting of Yin'), the place where Yin gathers. Balance is extremely
important in all Chi Kung systems, and development of the top must
be balanced by development of the bottom.

STRATEGY NOTE | *In the last three exercises, the practitioner has
mixed the Fire and Water with a bias towards the Water. This of
course balances the upward bias of the beginning exercises.*

2.8 | ENERGY TO THE NOSE

IT IS INTERESTING to note that almost all the inhalations and
exhalations in the system modulate the air with the nose with the
tip of the nose slightly contracted. Ancient Taoists believed that the
first energy to form in the body was the Ming Men and the first cells
were those of the nose. The tip of the nose was thought to be directly
related to the Ming Men. In the present day practice of acupuncture,
the tip of the nose can be used to treat the spine and acute lumbar
sprain (Ming Men area). It is also used to restore consciousness.
The point is able to redirect the route of elimination of liver toxins
to the lungs thus making exhalations more effective as cleansing
strategies.

Hua Shan Taoist Chi Kung emphasizes the importance of the tip of
the nose (GV 25) more than any other system that I am aware of.
As stated above, we accent GV 25 in most of our exercises. Recent
studies have shown that GV 25 is superior to GV 26 in reviving
consciousness.

GV 26 is located between the nose and the mouth (between Heaven and Earth). It has long been viewed as the most important point on the body for re-establishing Yin/Yang harmony to revive consciousness. GV 26 is associated with the Governing Vessel, Yang and the nose ('Gateway to Heavens Chi') and is also associated with the mouth, which receives the Essences from Earth. It is therefore between Heaven and Earth, Yin and Yang (represented by the Governing Vessel and the Conception Vessel).

Despite the fact that GV 26 is not the end point of the Governing Vessel (physical location for linking), the "between Heaven and Earth" energetics of the point provide a powerful linking of the Governing Vessel with the Conception Vessel. The point is also used to calm the mind through the Governing Vessel link to both the brain and the Heart.

Our system of Chi Kung uses GV 25 as the link between the Governing Vessel and the Conception Vessel, probably due to its link with the Ming Men ("remember the Governing Vessel and the Conception Vessel are the Yang and the Yin of the Ming Men"). It is interesting to note that in the nose microsystem of acupoints, the tip of the nose is related to the Kidneys, storehouse of the basic Yin and Yang of the body.

In Yoga, "gazing at the tip of the nose" with the two side channels unmoving (mental or physical) is said to directly awaken the Kundalini. The exercise brings the power up the Central Channel to Ajna Chakra where the inner light of the 'Essence of Being' appears.

To perform the Nose exercise, the practitioner Gathers the Energy in the Lower Tan Tien from a seated position. He then simply performs a long slow inhale while concentrating on the tip of the nose. The exercise ends with a Half Basic and a Basic and is repeated a total of five times.

STRATEGY NOTE | *Energy to the Nose addressed the area of meeting between the Conception Vessel and the Governing Vessel on the top of the body and Energy to the Genitals addressed the area of meeting at the bottom of the body. Addressing these two areas facilitates the harmonious linking of the two vessels in Little Earth and provides a safety valve for the exercising of the individual vessels as follows.*

2.9 | YIN PULSE (CONCEPTION VESSEL)

THE CONCEPTION VESSEL originates in the lower abdomen with the Governing Vessel and Chong Mai and emerges in the perineum. It ascends the midline of the body through the abdomen, chest, throat and jaw where it internally branches around the mouth and connects with the Governing vessel, continuing bilaterally to end below the eyes. Another branch extends from the lower abdomen, enters the spine, and rises up the back.

The Conception Vessel, called the 'Sea of the Yin Meridians,' is in charge of all the Yin of the body. It ensures the proper distribution of all the essences, blood and fluids that nourish life. The Conception Vessel performs these functions both for the life we have, and in the case of pregnancy, for the new life within. In both cases it protects and nourishes, extending the primal blueprint from the Source and regulating postnatal nourishment.

It is interesting to note that both 'Seas of Chi' are located on the Conception Channel, reinforcing the need for the interpenetration of Yin and Yang at every level. Reflecting this need for interpenetration, the internal channel of the Conception Vessel rises inside the spine, a major Yang area.

The exercise Yin Pulse is performed seated and repeated six times. Beginning with the nose, the Lower Tan Tien, Chong Mai and the genital points are linked in a downward progression. The exercise ends with a Half Basic and a Basic. It is generally acknowledged that opening the Conception Vessel is more difficult than opening the Governing Vessel.

2.10 | YANG PULSE (GOVERNING VESSEL)

THE GOVERNING VESSEL controls all the Yang of the body and is usually viewed as the channel that ascends through the spine to the brain ('Sea of Marrow'). A closer study of the vessel reveals that it actually has three branches. The first originates in the lower abdomen, descends to the perineum and genitals, ascends the interior of the spinal column and enters the Kidneys. The second branch originates in the lower abdomen, descends to the external genitalia, ascends to the umbilicus, Heart, and throat, winds around the mouth and terminates below the middle of the eyes. The final branch emerges at the inner canthus, bilaterally follows the Urinary Bladder channel up the forehead to the vertex where the two channels enter the brain. This branch emerges at Du 16, divides again and descends on either side of the spine to enter the Kidneys. The Governing Vessel and the Conception Vessel are Yin and Yang projections towards the exterior of the vibrancy of Ming Men.

The ascending power of the Governing Vessel brings Yang energy and spiritual stimulation to the brain. This facilitates the proper functioning of the upper orifices of perception and the cognitive functions that allow adaptation to the external environment. With its numerous connections to other functions, the Governing Vessel controls the animation of the entire body. It is sometimes referred to as the 'Sea of the Yang Meridians.'

The Governing Vessel is actually a mediator between the brain and the Heart. In texts on Chinese Medicine and Taoist Alchemy, Spirit is often mentioned both in reference to the Heart and the brain. The Heart is said to "house the spirit" and the Upper Tan Tien (brain) is called 'Spirit House.' This linking of brain and Heart by the Governing Vessel substantiates both views in their proper context.

To perform the Yang Pulse, the practitioner first Gathers Energy in the Lower Tan Tien, then directs that energy to the upper back and top of the head and ends the exercise with a Half Basic and a Basic. The process is repeated a total of nine times.

2.11 | LITTLE EARTH (MICROCOSMIC ORBIT)

LITTLE EARTH is the joining of the Conception and Governing Vessels in one smooth circular flow of energy. It is a common practice (techniques vary) with most systems of Chi Kung and considered mandatory for higher development.

Little Earth joins all the animating energies of Yang with all the nourishing energies of Yin to balance and nourish our "lives." Yang is said to have "no form" and Yin is said to have "form." For the Yang to function effectively, Yin must be present and for the Yin to be able to present itself as form, Yang must be present.Yin and Yang, form and function, are inescapably interconnected in every aspect of our existence.

The joining of the Conception Vessel and the Governing Vessel is both an opportunity to progress towards Divinity and a safety net to balance those powerful latent energies that will be brought into play through advanced Chi Kung training.

Little Earth exercises in Taoist Chi Kung are used to develop, store, and transform various energies to improve health and facilitate development. Opening these two channels is said to be a pre-requisite for opening the other six Extra-Meridians and, in fact, some authorities believe that all channels in the body will spontaneously open if the Little Earth is fully functioning. The fully functioning Governing and Conception Vessels are thought to gather energy from inside the body via various glandular se-cretions and from the environment. With the ability to gather and transform energy, the possibilities are unlimited.

Some systems of Taoist Chi Kung use the Little Earth as a vehicle for more advanced practices of specifically balancing vari-ous systems of the body and gathering environmental energies from both Heaven and Earth. It is also used in various sexual practices between men and women to help balance and replete Yin and Yang energies.

The Hua Shan Taoist Chi Kung Little Earth practice begins at the nose and progressively links the points of the Lower Tan Tien, Chong Mai, Genitals, Upper Back and Top of the Head. This cycle would be one revolution and the goal is to do nine revolutions. Our version is somewhat unusual in that all nine revolutions are done after only one initial inhale. The exercise ends with a Half Basic and a Basic.

STRATEGY NOTE | *This exercise has brought many of the preceding preparatory exercises together in our version of the famous Microcosmic Orbit. As you can see, some exercises from Level 1 are used to complete Little Earth including Double Breathing, Energy to the Upper Back and Shoulders and Energy Flow to the Top.*

2.12 | THE BEAR

THE BEAR is used to clear the Kidneys. "The Kidneys store Essence and dominate reproduction, growth and development. They produce marrow, dominate the bones, fill the brain (the brain is called the 'Sea of Marrow') and assist in blood production. Kidneys also control water and the reception of Chi." —*see pg. 45*

In Chinese Medicine, the Lungs inhale air, but the Kidneys "root" that air in the body. The Kidneys are the storehouse of energy for the body, and in some traditions are never directly cleaned. It is considered dangerous to take anything out of the Kidneys directly as this might cause a loss of "good" energy along with the "bad."

The Kidneys belong to the Water Element and are home to the Ming Men. Techniques in the Level 2 category bring Fire and Water together to "refine" energy. The benefits of this process give us access to high vibration "refined" energy capable of engendering good health and promoting Spiritual growth.

The dangers of bringing these two Elements together in an unbalanced manner are reversal of good health and Spiritual growth. When Fire and Water mix properly, "steam" is produced. If the mixture involves too much Water, the Fire can be put out and if Fire is in excess the Water can be burned up. Excess Fire is a common pitfall at this Level of training because Fire is by nature hot and the product of mixing ("steam") is also hot. A balanced system of Chi Kung will provide safeguards to protect both Water and Fire.

The Bear clears the Kidneys of excess from any cause. At this level of training, the Kidneys will naturally hold on to the good energy and allow the bad energy to be expelled. Since the Kidneys control the marrow (especially the spinal cord and brain), this exercise will eliminate toxin from those areas.

This exercise is obviously in the same genre of the early exercises from Level 1. At this stage of training, it is considered both safe and prudent to clean the Kidneys.

To perform the Bear, the practitioner raises his hands to the level of the head while inhaling. He then steps forward with his right leg, bends over placing his fists below the right knee while strongly "bowing" the spine and makes the cleansing sound for the Kidneys. Returning to standing, he finishes the exercise with a Basic.

2.13 | ENERGY DOWN BACK OF LEGS TO TOES

THE ORGAN that provides Yin/Yang balance for the Kidney in the Water element is the Urinary Bladder. The Urinary Bladder Channel is the longest channel in the body, running from the inner canthus of the eye, over the head, down the back and legs to terminate on the little toe. Branches of the channel enter the brain and its divergent channel enters the Heart.

The main functions of the Urinary Bladder are to store fluids and transform waste into urine for expulsion. It controls the quantity and quality of liquids in the body. Activating the cleansing function of the Urinary Bladder Channel is another important safety technique in Hua Shan Taoist Chi Kung.

Energy Down the Back of Legs to the Toes activates the whole
Urinary Bladder Channel, but especially the lower trajectory. Two
important points on the channel that are utilized for cleaning are
UB 39 and UB 40. Located behind the knees, both these points
are strongly activated by the exercise.

UB 39 is closely associated with the Triple Burner, Kidneys and
Urinary Bladder. It specifically acts on the transforming functions
of the Urinary Bladder. It has the ability to both remove excess
and strengthen function in the Lower Burner.

UB 40 is a powerful acupoint used to treat both urinary problems
and clear heat from the blood. Some authorities believe UB 40 is a
storage place for energy generated from meditation and that energy supports soul travel outside the body. This is one of the reasons
many Taoists do not sit cross-legged in meditation.

Another important result of this exercise is the activation of KI 1.
"The Yang channels of the legs carry energy from the body to the
feet. The only acupoint on the sole of the foot is KI 1. KI 1, referred
to as 'Gushing Spring' or 'Earth Surge,' is the place where the
energies of Earth and Man conjoin. It is an important point in balancing the body and absorbing energy from the Earth to support
the body's own energy."—*see Energy to the Soles, exercise 1.17, pg.
62*

This point can also help balance our bodies by draining toxins
into the ground.

Energy Down Back of Legs to Toes is performed by Gathering
Energy in the Lower Tan Tien, tensing the back of the legs and
drawing the energy downward. The exercise ends with a Half
Basic and a Basic.

STRATEGY NOTE | *The previous two exercises both energize
important areas of the body and provide a safety valve to allow
any unbalanced energies resulting from previous work or conditions to be dissipated.*

FOX IN A TREE utilizes the Governing Vessel (*see Yang Pulse*) and the Yang Chiao Mai (*see Yin/Yang Heel Pulse, exercise 2.36, pg. 145*) to harmonize the entire energy of the body. The exercise strengthens the back and legs, increases general circulation and balances blood pressure both high and low.

Early warning signs of incorrect energetic practices include an enlarged abdomen and high blood pressure. If the Water and Fire are not mixed properly and sufficient safeguards not observed, stagnation and/or blood pressure problems can result. This indicates a problem with Yang Energy.

Both the Governing Vessel and Yang Chiao Mai are related to Yang Energy. The Governing Vessel controls the Yang of the entire body and Yang Chiao Mai controls the movement and rhythms of Yang. Both vessels directly relate to the head. Yang Chiao Mai begins in the middle of the heel, thus is "rooted" in earth energy. These two vessels are often paired in acupuncture practice because they powerfully augment each other.

The "control" point of the Governing Vessel is SI 3, located on the ulnar side of the hand just proxipial to the head of the fifth metacarpal bone. Besides opening the Governing Vessel, it is used for treating upper back, neck and occipital problems. SI 3 also clears wind and heat and calms the Spirit.

Located directly below the lateral malleolus, UB 62 is the "control" point of Yang Chiao Mai. Besides opening the Yang Chiao Mai, UB 62 dispels both internal and external wind and calms the Spirit.

Stroke is a "wind" problem according to Chinese Medicine. As you can see, both points are indicated in "wind" conditions and have powerful effects on the Spirit (residing in the head).

After Gathering Energy in the Lower Tan Tien, performing Fox in a Tree requires the physical joining of SI 3 and UB 62. At this point another inhale is taken to balance the energy in both the

Lower Tan Tien and the Middle Tan Tien. Thereafter, either 9 or 12 steps are taken to "pump" the channels-creating balance in the energy flows. The exercise ends with a Half Basic and a Basic.

2.15 | DIAPHRAGM 2

I LIKE TO CALL Diaphragm 2 the "Great Harmonizer" because it so powerfully harmonizes Fire and Water (top and bottom).

The exercise starts similar to the Hawk in Level 1. "The exercise begins with the practitioner bent 90° at the waist with arms hanging down and hands in fists. He stands up inhaling while spreading the arms to the sides at shoulder level (bringing energy up in the body and expanding the chest)."—*see Hawk, exercise 1.5, pg. 45*. Then after swallowing to the Lower Tan Tien, the practitioner bends parallel to the ground and makes the POOH sound.

While performing a long slow inhale, the practitioner moves first to the left and then to the right bending one leg and extending the other while turning the waist from side to side so that the arms are perpendicular over each knee. Movements go to each side three times and the exercise ends with a Half Basic and a Basic.

From a mechanical point of view, the Two Side Channels are activated by the side to side stretching. The outspread arms and twisting waist energize both the Lower Tan Tien (low back and Kidneys) and the Middle Tan Tien (chest and diaphragm), Fire and Water are mixed by the breathing strategy, filling the Lower Tan Tien with energy, then continuing to inhale energy through the Middle Tan Tien to the Lower Tan Tien. The legs play an important role in the overall function of Diaphragm 2.

The bi-lateral trajectory of the Gall Bladder Meridian runs from head to toe on both sides of the body. By alternately expanding and contracting the Gall Bladder Meridian through the side to side leg movements, that Meridian is heavily activated. The Gall Bladder Meridian is the main source of energy for the Belt Channel.

The Belt Channel literally circles the waist like a belt. It has the function of binding all the vertical channels of the body together in general, and specifically accesses the Kidney, Liver, Spleen, Conception Vessel, Chong Mai, and according to Chi Kung theory the Governing Vessel via Ming Men (GV 4).

This binding function not only holds the other channels, but also harmonizes and unifies them. By exerting the proper amount of pressure, the Belt Channel regulates the upward and downward flows of energy in the other channels, thus harmonizing the upper and lower body.

The Gall Bladder itself is activated by energizing its meridian. The Gall Bladder is Yin/Yang paired with the Liver. The Liver energy represents a tremendous springing up and expansion of life energy. The Gall Bladder energy is the force that focuses that upsurging energy into correct expression. This is why the Gall Bladder is associated with correct decision making and why it is used to "correct" the expression of our refined energy. Being an expression of the Wood Element (first expansion of life force from the Source), Gall Bladder energy is closely linked to the Ming Men, source of our transformations.

The Gall Bladder stands out among the Yang organs as the only one that "stores" essences. The other Yang Organs are involved in the digestive cycle, transporting and processing but not "storing." Since the essences are the clearest result of the digestive process from which our correct form will express itself, the "correctness" of the Gall Bladder can be utilized by those pure substances.

2.16 | MOUTH—BACK OF NECK TO TOES

THIS EXERCISE concentrates energy in the 'Jade Pillow,' a point at the base of the skull. This point functions as a pump to draw energy up the spine, as a link to the cerebellum and medulla oblongata (which control respiration, heartbeat, muscle co-ordination, etc.) and as a storage depot for refined energy. Some authorities believe this point resonates with Yin energies to help balance the Yang of the head. It is also said to be an area of receptivity of Divine information.

'Jade Pillow' is one of the three important gates on the spine that need to be opened to nourish the brain. It is directly connected to the crown (GV 20) and First Tan Tien (third Eye). The importance of working on this point as refined energy begins to circulate in the body cannot be underestimated.

Mouth-Back of Neck to Toes gathers energy from several sources including the Governing Vessel, Two Side Channels, and Yang Wei Mai. The energy is brought up to Jade Pillow to open and energize the point and then circulated back down to the toes to nourish and balance the whole body.

After Gathering the Energy in the Lower Tan Tien, 'Jade Pillow' is activated by body position and mental focus while performing a long slow inhale. The energy is then directed down the body to the toes while exhaling slowly but steadily. The exercise ends with a Basic.

STRATEGY NOTE | *The previous three exercises are instrumental in balancing and harmonizing the energies of the upper and lower body.*

2.17 | RETURN THE HORMONE

THE TITLE "Return the Hormone" refers to the main function of this exercise, which is to replete the Kidneys/Lower Tan Tien. The Kidneys (including sex organs and adrenals in Chinese Medicine) produce powerful hormones that have far-reaching effects on our health and provide "fuel" for our Spiritual growth.

Adrenaline, testosterone, and estrogen affect the energy levels in the body, the sexual/reproductive function, and in proper amounts delay aging. The levels of testosterone and estrogen in the body are directly proportional with the level of growth hormone.

Growth hormone decline is a major indication of aging. Growth hormone promotes both fat burning and muscle building in the body. Decline in this hormone adversely affects body composition, immune function and coronary health as well as a host of other age related conditions.

Although growth hormone is produced in the Pituitary Gland (more the province of Level 3 exercises), Taoists believe that supporting any aspect of the endocrine system helps all aspects. They believe the seven main glands in the body—sexual glands, adrenals, pancreas, thymus, thyroid, pituitary, and pineal—form an interdependent chain of energetic potential through which we can activate our full evolvement.

After Gathering Energy in the Lower Tan Tien, the practitioner drops to a kneeling position and strongly "bows" his back. He then performs twelve waist-twisting rotations while lifting and circling his arms. Six of the rotations are accompanied by inhales and six are not. The exercise ends with a Half Basic and a Basic.

The waist turning stimulates the Kidneys, the arm movements draw energy up the Two Side Channels and the breathing strategy strengthens both Yin and Yang aspects of the Kidneys. The physical position and breath strategy unite the Fire and Water.

2.18 | ENERGY IN A BOTTLE

ENERGY IN A BOTTLE is designed to replete the Middle Tan Tien and connect it to the Lower Tan Tien. In this exercise, the body is filled with energy.

After Gathering Energy in the Lower Tan Tien, the legs and upper back areas are filled with energy through successive inhales. The chest/Middle Tan Tien is then engorged with energy through eight more inhales accompanied by hand/arm motions that direct the energy from the Lower Tan Tien to the Middle Tan Tien completely filling the Middle Tan Tien. In this case, we are bringing the Water to the Fire and expanding the Fire.

2.19 | ENERGY IN THE BLADDER

ENERGY IN THE BLADDER circulates the refined energy from the previous two exercises throughout the body.

The Urinary Bladder Meridian extends from the inner canthus of the eyes, traverses the head, back, and posterior leg and ends in the little toe. Along its length are points that affect every tissue and organ in the body. Connecting with both the Kidneys and the Urinary Bladder, it is ideally suited to disperse refined energy throughout the body.

The general functions of the Urinary Bladder are to store liquids, separate the clear from the turbid and convert the turbid to urine. More than simply storing fluids, the Urinary Bladder organizes the fluids of the body. Through this organization, the transformations of Chi are able to appropriately manifest. It creates a stage upon which the transformed Chi can act by clearly delineating and regulating the pathways of Water.

Energy in the Bladder is a simple exercise. After Gathering energy in the Tan Tien, the practitioner inhales again and with body and mind concentrates energy in the Bladder. The exercise ends with a Half Basic and a Basic.

It should be noted that the misuse of Bladder energy is one of the main dangers of energetic practices. The results of this misuse include a large abdomen and high blood pressure (especially after age 50). The cause of disharmony in the Bladder is energy misdirected and stagnated. When activating the Lower Tan Tien, it is not enough to simply "gather, hold or direct" energy to the lower abdomen as is often recommended. The precise methods of directing and the proper destinations of this energy must be understood by each practitioner in order for him to safely gain any benefit from such practices.

Concentrating on energy gathering in the lower abdomen is a common practice that martial artists utilize to develop power. Done properly great power can be generated and stored with these techniques. Great power can manifest even if the techniques are done improperly but in the long run that power will exact a heavy payment.

2.20 | HEART AND KIDNEY MEET INSIDE

HEART AND KIDNEY Meet Inside is a surgically precise energetic masterpiece for bringing Fire and Water together at their most subtle expressions. The old classics state that it is important to bring the essences (innermost parts) of Fire and Water together to produce the true refined energy ('the Golden Elixir').

The Heart/Fire represents the Middle Tan Tien and the Kidneys/ Water represent the Lower Tan Tien. The hexagrams representing Fire and Water are:

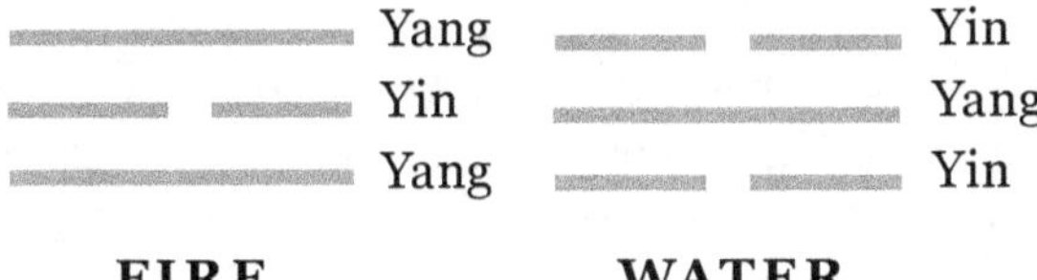

The middle line of the Fire trigram is a Yin line representing the original Water from which Fire came, and the middle line of the Water trigram is a Yang line representing the original Fire.

As you will remember from the Five Element Diagram (*see pg. 10*), each organ/meridian is associated with one of the Five Elements. The Heart is associated with the Fire Element and the Kidneys with the Water Element. Each of the Elements is represented on every one of the Twelve Regular Meridians by a point corresponding to the individual Element. For example, the Heart has one point representing Fire, one representing Earth, one representing Metal, one representing Water and one representing Wood.

In Heart and Kidney Meet Inside, attention on the Water point of the Heart Meridian is used to draw the original Water from the Heart. After Collecting Energy in the Lower Tan Tien, this drawing out of the Water is accomplished through inhaling while moving energy from the Heart to its Water point. The Water point of the Heart is then connected to the front gathering point of the Kidneys and the Heart/Water energy is exhaled into the Kidney point. Next, the Heart/Water energy is drawn from the Kidney gathering point into the Kidney and the Kidney/Fire energy is drawn up to the Heart. The exercise ends with a Half Basic and a Basic.

The philosophical trigram representation of the new "refined" state is

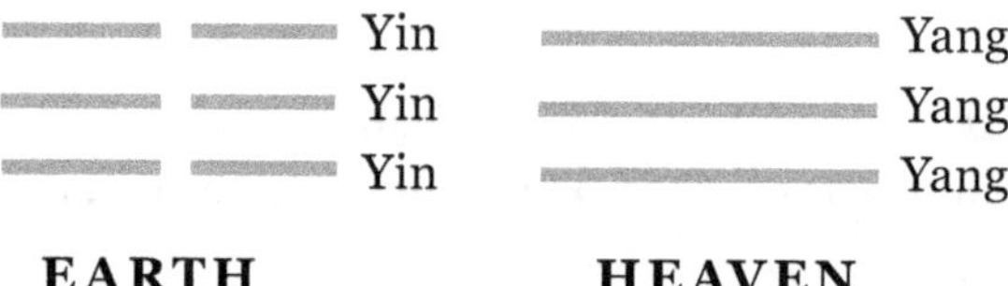

Philosophically, macrocosmic (the universe) balance hinges on Heaven and Earth and microcosmic (man) balance hinges on Fire and Water. The result of this exercise is to bring man back into harmony with the unlimited universal energies from which he was created.

2.21 | LONG BREATHING

LONG BREATHING is the first exercise of the meditative side of Hua Shan Taoist Chi Kung. In Level 2, there are two so called "sitting practices." Level 3 has several more "sitting practices" and continued involvement in the system will reveal a large number of meditative techniques.

Countless volumes have been written on meditations from many different disciplines. One could spend a lifetime trying to understand the intricacies of the mind and still not acquire development. As with Chi Kung, the only way to get the benefit from meditation is to meditate. Nevertheless, there are some interesting things to note in regards to "sitting practices."

The mind, breath and energies of the body are intricately linked. Movement in one will produce responding movement in the others. Likewise stillness in one will induce stillness in the others. Each meditation induces a particular energy flow and breath rhythm in the body. Conversely, controlling the breath and/or energy flows in the body can affect the mind. Sitting practices are usually not emphasized in Hua Shan Chi Kung until the energy flows smoothly and easily in the body, facilitating the effects of meditation.

The two sitting practices in Level 2 work on the breath and mind. Long Breathing accents breath regulation and Quiet Sitting works on stilling the mind. One of the points of contention between various factions of the spiritual community is which works best—regulating breath or regulating mind. In this system we have numerous techniques for both. In fact, regulations of mind, breath and energies are involved directly or indirectly in most sitting practices and, of course, there is always the highest sitting of "no regulation."

The mind acts like a "wild horse or monkey" being difficult to keep from pursuing multiple thoughts. By quieting the breath, the mind can be quieted.

The breath is directly influenced by the central nervous system and brain. Disturbed breathing patterns affect the brain and nervous system, and vice versa. We are all familiar with the effects of emotional disharmonies of all types on breathing patterns. Through the nervous system, disharmony in any area of the body can affect breath. Breath, in return, can affect every area of the body and the mind.

The technique for Long Breathing is simple. While seated comfortably (spine straight and not touching anything with feet flat on the floor), the practitioner Gathers Energy in the Lower Tan Tien and directs half that energy to the upper back. He then begins to take long, slow, deep, fine breaths. The inhale is longer than the exhale by a particular ratio.

By inhaling longer than exhaling (as in Walking Chi Kung), energy is actually gathered into the body through this exercise. The feet are flat on the ground to create balance through KI 1. The exercise ends with a Basic.

2.22 | DEVELOP THE STOMACH

AT FIRST SIGHT, Develop the Stomach does not appear to fit very well in Level 2. It is a simple exercise, seemingly devoid of "heavy" energetic mixings. With a deeper look at the forces at work, the importance of this exercise becomes apparent. It functions to both unite Fire and Water and also to offer support to the processes set in motion by Level 2.

The Stomach and Spleen (*see Thinking Energy, exercise 2.27, pg. 138*)) represent the Earth Element, dominate the Middle Heater (center) and control the upward and downward movements of the digestive process in the body. They are in charge of storehouses and granaries and as such, essential for the continuation of life. The energetic function of storehouses and granaries is to "receive and distribute." Both Fire and Water energy, in passing through the center, are "received and distributed." Some authorities believe the actual mixing takes place in the Middle Burner.

There is another important function for both Develop the Stomach (Stomach) and Thinking Energy (Spleen). In Chapter 2 (pg. 29), we mentioned the crest of Chi flowing through the Twelve Regular Meridians. The crest flows through each meridian in a two hour period, thus with twelve meridians the cycle completes itself in twenty-four hours. This is reflected in the following chart:

THE TIMES ARE:

Lung: 3—5 am | Large Intestine: 5—7 am | Stomach: 7—9 am
Spleen: 9—11 am | Heart: 11 am—1 pm | Small Intestine: 1—3 pm
Urinary Bladder: 3—5 pm | Kidney: 5—7 pm
Pericardium: 7—9 pm | Triple Burner: 9—11 pm
Gall Bladder: 11 pm—1 am | Liver: 1—3 am

According to the Midday/Midnight Theory, organs on the opposite sides of this "clock" have a direct relationship to each other. In other words, the Stomach: 7—9 am is directly related to the Pericardium: 7—9 pm and the Spleen: 9—11 am is directly related to the Triple Burner: 9—11 pm.

The Pericardium and Triple Burner are involved in all the transformations of Fire and Water in the body. By working on the Stomach and Spleen in Level 2, we support all the other transformations, and of course by harmonizing Earth we increase the safety of the whole process.

After Swallowing Energy to the Lower Tan Tien, the practitioner inhales through the mouth directly into the stomach. By body position, he first squeezes the stomach closed and then opens it during the inhale. This has the function of first drawing energy up from the Stomach and then pulling energy down into the Stomach —up from below (Water) and down from above (Fire). The exercise ends with a Half Basic and a Basic.

STRATEGY NOTE | *Thinking Energy (see exercise 2.27, pg. 138) is the other exercise for this strategy of harmonizing the Middle Burner.*

2.23 | EYES CAN LOOK AT SUN

THIS EXERCISE is performed as a safety procedure for the Sun part of Gathering the Essence of the Sun and Moon. It engorges the eyeballs with Chi and Blood to protect them from the rays of the Sun. Since the Liver corresponds to the eyes, Eyes Can Look At Sun also stimulates Liver function.

After Gathering Energy in the Lower Tan Tien, the eyes are massaged by pressing the inner border, the outer border, the whole eyes and finally rubbing the eyes from inner to outer borders. The exercise ends with a Basic.

2.24 | WALKING CHI KUNG

WALKING CHI KUNG is designed to mix the Fire and Water in the body and to add energy from the environment to that mix. The practitioner Gathers Energy in the Lower Tan Tien then proceeds to walk twelve steps with his arms spread wide (to open the chest (Middle Tan Tien) both for drawing Water energy up to meet the Fire and to collect environmental energy). These twelve steps are accompanied by inhaling to the chest.

After completing the inhale period, the practitioner places his fists at the lower abdomen and walks six steps exhaling to the Lower Tan Tien. This brings the mixed energy from the Middle Tan Tien to the Lower Tan Tien.

The walking continues for as long as desired, all the while mixing Fire and Water and gathering environmental energy to augment the energies of the body. The exercise ends with a Basic.

STRATEGY NOTE | *Walking exercises are an important part of Chi Kung Practices from many lineages. Walking itself is an enormously beneficial exercise and has been well represented in "health literature." Aside from the physical attributes of the exercise, walking often enables people to get out of their usual environment and experience nature. That experience alone would make walking beneficial.*

One of the benefits seldom mentioned by western authors is the enhanced energy circulation promoted by walking. Chi Kung exercises utilize change in the body to open the channels and spark increases in circulation and transformation. Philosophically this change is represented by the alternate emphasis on Yin and Yang, the polar opposites. In Chi Kung exercises, this philosophy is manifested through many opposites including fast and slow, hard and soft, high and low, inside and outside, inhale and exhale, etc.

By its nature, walking promotes change. The back and forth motion of the limbs and, especially the alternation of weight bearing on the legs, profoundly affects circulation in the body. By adding various breath and mind regulations to the basic form, or changing the basic form to direct and increase change, walking becomes a powerful tool for health and transformation.

2.25 | TAN TIEN SAME AS LUNG

TAN TIEN SAME as Lung is the only "sleep" exercise in our system. The goal of the exercise is not to work with dreams, as is sometimes done with other lineages. This system aspires to dreamless sleep, allowing the mind to be as inactive as possible. Occasionally inspired dreams can grace the sleeping state, but our system aims at emptying and quieting the mind when asleep. The exercise is said to make the practitioner "breath like he did in the womb" all night.

This exercise does not "Gather" at the beginning nor end with a Basic. The practitioner, by body position and intense reverse breathing, activates the union of Fire and Water just before he falls asleep. The result is a little like stoking the fire in a woodstove heated house at the end of the day. A well-stoked fire will keep the house warm all night.

The intense, reverse breathing in this exercise stimulates the circulation of energy and fluids in the spine and brain. Tan Tien Same as Lung alternately pressurizes and depressurizes the brain, creating rhythmic energy flows that clear the mind and induce harmony.

The pumping action of the diaphragm stimulates the Lungs, Heart and digestive organs and clears the sinuses. This helps eliminate stagnations that may disturb sleep.

Successful practice of Tan Tien Same as Lung insures smooth circulation in the body all night literally keeping the practitioner warm as well as allowing for further refinement during sleep.

2.26 | FOUR BREATHING

FOUR BREATHING is the next progression up from Double Breathing and Three Breaths of Energy: as described in the Level 1 exercises. Like those exercises, it promotes circulation in the body and energizes the particular areas addressed by the exercise.

The next progression is Five Breathing (*see Five Breathing, exercise 2.29, pg. 139*). A more in-depth discussion of all four of these exercises will be presented with that exercise.

Four Breathing is performed the same way as Three Breaths of Energy, except another breath is added to fill the lower part of the body.

2.27 | THINKING ENERGY

THE UNDERLYING THEORY of Thinking Energy has already been discussed with Develop the Stomach (*see Develop the Stomach, exercise 2.22, pg. 134*). This exercise directs refined energy from mixing Fire and Water to each of the four limbs. As you will remember from Level 1, the Spleen controls the energy in the four limbs. Both Develop the Stomach (Stomach) and Thinking Energy (Spleen) have a strong impact on digestive energy which is fundamental for health and evolution.

Thinking Energy is actually performed as four separate exercises. Each part has a Gathering Energy in the Lower Tan Tien beginning and ends with a Half Basic and a Basic. The individual parts each bring Fire energy from the Middle Tan Tien to Water energy in the Lower Tan Tien and then directs the energy refined through that mixing to one of the limbs. The direction of the energy is accomplished both through the concentration of the mind and through specific body regulation.

2.28 | CHANGE OLD AIR FOR NEW

CHANGE OLD AIR FOR NEW, is another cleansing exercise. It is recommended to do this exercise three times upon arising in the morning and once in the evening.

During the night, despite the good effects of Tan Tien Same As Lung, energy tends to stagnate in the body due to lack of physical movement. Stagnation impedes the smooth flow of energy, which is one of the primary concerns of Chi Kung practice. By changing the "air" in the morning, the body can be cleaned and revitalized.

In regards to "cleaning," an effective Tan Tien Same as Lung exercise may well continue to clean the body as we sleep. Eliminating any waste dislodged during the night is an important consideration in the morning.

Eliminating toxins accumulated during the day is also important. Because we are much more physically active during the daytime (physical activity helps move energy and clean the body), the exercise can be effective with only one repetition.

After Gathering Energy in the Lower Tan Tien, the practitioner performs a slightly different version of the first movement of the Basic, gathering any toxins or stagnations at the level of the chest. Then, using the clearing sound of the Heart, he squeezes his body down while performing the last motion of the Basic. After repeating this process six times, he ends with a Basic.

The sound for the Heart, according to ancient texts, is capable of cleaning the whole body.

2.29 | FIVE BREATHING

FIVE BREATHING is the last exercise in the genre of exercises activating the specific five body areas (and therefore the Five Elements). Five Breathing adds the head to the areas addressed by Four Breathing. A common saying in the Taoist Chi Kung community is "Five Chi go to the Source."

Yoga has the five Vayus -upward moving Vayu, downward moving Vayu, middle moving Vayu, left moving Vayu and right moving Vayu. The Chinese Medical Community and Chi Kung Community have the Five Elements. In both traditions, the basic number of distinct energies is recognized as five. From these five energies that evolved from the basic dual polarity, spring all the functions that organize and animate our being.

One of the signs said to represent the successful conversion of Jing to Chi, or the cultivation of the Chi Level, is the repleting of the energy levels of the Five Chi, organically represented by the Heart/upward moving/head, Kidneys/downward moving/feet, Spleen/center moving/center, Liver/right moving/upper back, Lungs/left moving/chest. These energies are more subtle than the organ structures, hence they are not confined to either the physical locations or the sphere of influences of the organs.

Of course, it is important to have the five organs balanced and replete. Several Level 1 exercises are designed to accomplish this task. As higher and higher vibrational energy is expressed in the body through any energetic practice, it is important to have adequate development for handling that energy. Development takes time and work. As my teacher always says, "Nothing real is fast."

In Level 1, two exercises that address some of the five energies have already been called upon. To replete the middle moving and left moving energies we used Double Breathing and to replete the middle moving, right moving and left moving energies we used Three Breaths of Energy.

For the purposes of Level 1, middle moving energy/Earth/center represents the mother of all form. Left moving energy/Metal/chest represents the bringing to fruition and solidity of that form and right moving energy/wood/upper back represents growth and expansion.

Four Breathing adds repletion of the downward moving energy and Five Breathing repletes the upward moving energies.

Downward moving/Water and upward moving/Fire are added in Level 2 because they are more directly linked to the 'FIRE and WATER' from which the others sprang and are the special province of Level 2.

In Level 2, higher vibrational energies are generated and infused into the system. It is especially important that all five of the basic energies are replete and in communication with each other so that they can harmoniously interact. Disharmony and lack of communication between the five energies while the body/mind/spirit complex is exposed to this "refined" energy can lead to damage.

According to most authorities, 'Five Chi go to the Source' refers to the repletion of the original state of the five energies in both quantity and function. In Level 3, there is an exercise that actually returns the five energies to the Original Source through shutting off the senses.— *see Closing the Nine Holes, exercise 3.27, pg. 168*

2.30 | QUIET SITTING

QUIET SITTING is the "mind regulation" part of the Level 2 sitting practices. Basically, it involves assuming the same sitting position as Long Breathing then Gathering Energy in the Lower Tan Tien—moving half that energy to the upper back and sitting with no thoughts—good luck. This form of meditation is quite common and easy to research, if desired.

In the Taoist Chi Kung community the saying 'Three Flowers Meet at the Top' is also used in reference to the Chi Level. In Yoga circles, references are often made to the Two Side Channels and Central Channel meeting in the Brow Chakra (Upper Tan Tien for Taoists). The Three Flowers for Taoists are the Jing (Essence), Chi (Energy) and Shen (Spirit).

Basically, in either tradition, there would be a joining in the Upper Tan Tien before the movement to the top or crown. This is a different phenomenon than moving energy to or through the crown. "Three Flowers Meet at the Top" implies that "refinement" of Fire and Water and ascension through the Central Channel has occurred. This is certainly possible and is often a spontaneous occurrence when the polarities are joined.

Some authorities believe that the 'Five Chi go to the Source' happens at about the same time as Three Flowers Meet at the Top,' which is why it is spoken of as a gauge of Chi Level success. It is also one of the goals of Level 3 spirit practices.

In any case, if your Chi Level practice is bearing fruit, Quiet Sitting offers the opportunity for spontaneous unity of the Three Flowers.

STRATEGY NOTE | *As we know from the information presented in Level 1, the Heart controls the vessels. The vessels include all the networks of circulation in the body, including pathways of Blood and Chi.*

Blood and Chi are intimately related. They are both renewed from the transformation of food and liquids by the Spleen/Stomach. Although, coming from the same place, they have different natures. Chi has no form, is related to Yang, and functions as an animator and transformer. Blood has form, is related to Yin, and functions to nourish and to irrigate.

On the one hand, Blood is dependent upon Chi to transform substances, which are used to produce Blood. On the other hand, Blood is the vehicle through which Essences are made available for transformation, which results in Chi. In the body, Chi (Yang) needs Blood (Yin) to express itself, and Blood needs Chi for circulation and transformation. All these interactions take place through the circulation in the vessels. The terms Blood and Chi are often used to represent the overall interpenetration and balance of Yin and Yang in the body.

The Essences, carried by the Blood, hold and transport Spirits through the circulation of Blood. It is the Spirits (entering the Heart from Heaven) that orchestrate all the transformations in the body. It is at the level of the Blood/Chi that the Divine expresses itself to maintain all our functions.

The following two exercises open and support the veins and arteries of the body, which extend the influence of the Spirits throughout our form and support the functions of Fire.

2.31 | CIRCULATION IN THE VEINS

THIS EXERCISE increases circulation in the veins. After Gathering Energy in the Lower Tan Tien, the arms (with hands in Tiger Claws to open the chest) and legs are used to pump the body, utilizing alternating weight and tension shifts to mechanically energize the veins. Multiple inhales add energy from the outside to the system and facilitate the mixing of Fire and Water. The movements themselves activate the Two Side Channels, the Middle Tan Tien and the Lower Tan Tien.

2.32 | HOLD BREATHING

HOLD BREATHING addresses the arteries. The exercise consists of four parts which are modifications of the Monkey, Hawk, Turtle and Energy to the Upper Arms (all Level 1 exercises). Each part mimics its namesake from Level 1, except that when there are movements they are done four times rather than six (Hawk, Turtle, and Energy to Upper arms) and there is no breathing during the movements. In all four parts, the energy is held inside and moderate tension is expressed throughout the exercise thus increasing blood flow in the arteries.

2.33 | GATHER THE ESSENCE OF THE SUN AND MOON

MOST PRACTITIONERS of Taoist Systems of Chi Kung utilize energy from nature to augment and sometimes balance their own organic energy. Nature is a treasure chest of valuable energies for those who know how to access and absorb it. The sun, moon, trees, earth, sky, stars, animals, mountains, flowers, etc. all express powerful energies that are available to man.

In Level 2, Hua Shan Chi Kung practitioners learn to gather the energies of the sun and moon. The sun represents pure Yang Chi. Gathering this Yang Chi can help remove toxins from the body, tonify deficient Yang, consolidate the Source Chi and prevent premature aging. The moon represents pure Yin Chi. Gathering this Yin Chi can nourish the Kidneys, strengthen the essence, fortify the marrow, strengthen the brain, replete Yin deficiency, and contribute to longevity.

The techniques for gathering Sun and Moon Chi are identical. The practitioner uses his palms, eyes and mouth to swallow and guide Chi to his Lower Tan Tien. The technique is repeated six times and the exercise is repeated three times.

To gather the Sun Chi, one must first perform Eyes can Look at Sun (*see exercise 2.23, pg.135*) to protect his eyes. Then, just as the sun rises, the practitioner "gathers." It is also best to gather the moon at moonrise. These rising times get the chi while it is "growing."

Gathering the chi of the moon is most effective three days before and three days after the full moon. Since the sun and moon are in Yin/Yang balance, when the sun is at its best, the moon is at its worst, and vice versa. Therefore, the best time for gathering the sun is at the end of the moon's cycle.

2.34 | LONG STRONG BREATHING

LONG STRONG BREATHING is, perhaps, the most powerful Fire and Water mixer in Level 2. After Gathering Energy in the Lower Tan Tien, air from outside is inhaled into the lungs and energy from inside is brought up to the Middle Tan Tien from the Lower Tan Tien. This long, strong engorgement of the Middle Tan Tien is followed by a forceful exhale and descent of the energy in the Middle Tan Tien to the Lower Tan Tien (through body position and breath). The whole process is repeated two more times and the exercise ends with a Basic.

STRATEGY NOTE | *Long-Strong Breathing uses body position and breath control to force the Fire and Water together. The intended result of this Fire and Water mixing is that energy "refined" through the process will enter the Central Channel and rise to the head, spontaneously or through direction, depending on the technique to nourish the Spirit. Generally speaking, spontaneous ascensions are the province of Level 2 and directed ascensions are the province of Level 3 (Level 3 does not rule out spontaneous ascensions by any means).*

It is interesting to note that the next exercise, Inhale to Kidney, perfectly sets the stage for spontaneous ascension through the Central Channel and the last exercise, Yin/Yang Heel Pulse, opens other pathways to the brain.

2.35 | INHALE TO KIDNEY

AT FIRST APPEARANCE, Inhale to Kidney is a sitting version of Energy Flow to the Kidney from Level 1. Both exercises engorge the Kidneys with energy through breath, mind, and body position. It is a small adjustment in body position that accounts for their difference. In Energy Flow to the Kidneys, the head and neck are arched back to prevent the energy from rising. In Inhale to Kidney, the head is down, opening the spinal column and providing not only an open pathway to the head, but also internal pressure to "coax" refined energy into the Central Channel.

2.36 | YIN/YANG HEEL PULSE

THE NAME of this exercise refers to the Yin and Yang Chiao Mai, which are two of the Extra-Ordinary Channels that begin on the heels and meet deep in the brain.

The Yang Chiao Mai runs from the outer heels up the sides of the body and neck where it crosses the face to the inner canthus of the eye (where it joins the Yin Chiao Mai) and runs over the head to the rear where it enters the brain. Ordinarily, it is believed that it is nourished by Chi generated from exercising the legs and functions to regulate Yang.

The Yin Chiao Mai runs from the inner heels up the inside of the legs, ascends the abdomen and neck, crosses the face where it meets the Yang Chiao Mai at the inner canthus of the eye and enters the brain. It derives its Chi from an intimate connection with the Kidney Channel and the sex glands. In higher Chi Kung practices, this channel is engorged with energy which is directed upwards and used to nourish the Spirit (brain). The nourishment received by the Spirit from Yin Chiao Mai is one of the major factors contributing to "Enlightenment."

Some authorities believe that the two channels make a continuous loop of energy, with the Yin Chiao Mai bringing Ancestral Energy up to the head (after receiving it from the Kidney Channel in the heel) and the Yang Chiao Mai bringing Ancestral Energy back down to the feet.

The above information is usually what is expressed regarding these two channels, but a more detailed look at their functions reveals a more fascinating picture.

Both channels actually begin in the middle of the heel and meet in the depths of the brain. Their origin links them to the energies of the Earth, and their ending links them to Heaven through the brain/Spirit. They are the first bilateral channels, and through their pathways on the inside and outside of the body represent the communication of Yin and Yang at all levels of the body.

The Chiao Mai regulate the rhythms of Yin and Yang in the body, the ascending and descending on the left and the right. Medically, the Yin Chiao Mai is often used with the Conception Vessel and the Yang Chiao Mai is used with the Governing Vessel. Both Yin and Yang Chaio Mai and the Governing and Conception Vessels are ever circulating loops of Yin/Yang energy, concerned with co-penetration and balance.

Ancient texts refer to "breathing from the heels." The inference is that not only do we take in essences from Heaven through the Lungs, but also Earth essences through the heels. The Chiao channels provide both roots in the Earth whereby sustenance can be acquired and the impetus to move that sustenance upward into the body.

These two exercises are performed by Gathering Energy in the lower Tan Tien (Water), inhaling again to activate the Fire, mixing the two and, depending on the exercise, engorging either the Yin or Yang Chiao Mai. The exercises end with a Half Basic and a Basic.

STRATEGY NOTE | *It is interesting to note that the ending of the Level 2 exercises (which are concerned with moving the Yin and Yang back together) addresses the Chaio channels, which are the first Yin/Yang movement regulators in the body and are also an important link to the brain/Spirit which is the special province of Level 3 Exercises.*

This completes the thirty six exercises of Level 2. ☯

CHAPTER 10

Exercises for Level 3 | Shen

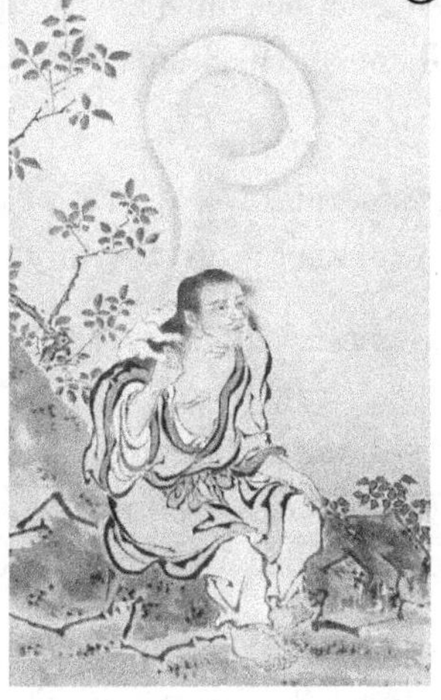

WHEN SPEAKING OF SHEN (Spirit) in relationship to Inner Alchemy, there are two general aspects that attract our attention.

The first aspect refers to our "mind" and covers the whole range of mental activities including all our thought and emotional processes. This aspect of Spirit is said to reside in the Heart and is responsible for our personality and the quality of our consciousness. Although, each of the Five Yin Organs houses some aspect of our "mind," it is the Heart that co-ordinates its overall activities, both conscious and sub-conscious. This "mind" is conditioned by its environment and is the source of those activities (ie. desire, attachment, expectation, etc.) that bring suffering to our lives. It is also a valuable tool for discerning the pathway to ultimate liberation.

This aspect of Shen (Spirit) is connected to the realm of the Five Elements, thus exercises in Level 1 (Essence) have a profound effect on the functions and balance of the "mind."

In fact, it is important to have a well integrated "mind" before activating the potential energies of Level 2 (Energy). The high vibrational energy activated in Level 2 exercises effect both the Essence and Spirit Levels.

At the level of Essence, Shen provides high quality healing and rejuvenating energies. These energies must have "open" pathways in the Essence Level to be utilized and avoid inappropriate results from its presence.

At the level of Spirit, the energies from Level 2 exercises nourish the potential for singularity (oneness with Divinity).

The second aspect of Shen refers to our Original Spirit, 'our direct link to the Divine.' This aspect is said to reside in the Upper Tan Tien, and its activation and nourishment is the province of Level 3 exercises. The Original Spirit is beyond conditioning and limit. Access to the Original Spirit increases "grace" in our lives and eventually leads us to that singularity.

The two aspects of Shen are interactive, with the "mind" aspect providing regulation of the body/mind complex and providing the information for the pathway to "refinement" while the Original Spirit links the microcosm of "self" to the macrocosm of "singularity."

Exercises in Level 3 are basically designed to energize the brain with refined energy from Level 2 transformations. The Little Earth Orbit, Central Channel (Chong Mai) and the Yin/Yang Chiao Mai channels are the main pathways that transport this "refined" energy to the brain.

There are two other areas addressed by Level 3 exercises. The first is the extension of the practitioners consciousness/Spirit beyond the physical confines of his body, either to gather highly potent energies from nature to supplement his own energies or to return to "singularity." The second is to direct energy circulation into the deepest levels of the body symbolized by and manifested in the "bones." 'Marrow Washing' (bone energy circulation) is considered necessary to attain the highest levels of Chi Kung practice.

Various exercises to activate energies in the feet are also included in Level 3. These support and balance the upward thrust of many of the other exercises, as well as open the connection between Man and Earth.

3.1 | HAWK INHALING

HAWK INHALING is designed to mix the Fire and Water through focusing the breathing alternately in the chest (inhaling) and the Lower Tan Tien (exhaling). "Flapping the arms" increases the movement of energy between the two areas and the stances (one leg bent and the other straight with toes pointed up) open the two Chiao Vessels which augment energy flow to the brain. The mixing of Fire and Water automatically activates the Two Side Channels (Ming Men) thereby stimulating the Central Channel (Chong Mai) and the Little Earth. This exercise dramatically increases energy flow to the head through the Central Channel, the Chiao Mai and Little Earth.

3.2 | TAI CHI WALKING (DWARF WALKING)

THIS EXERCISE is commonly practiced by Wu Style Tai Chi players (known as 'cat walking') without the emphasis on the breath. It is excellent for encouraging the harmonious interactions of Yin and Yang in the body and in advanced practices can be used to gather energy from the Earth. Again, the position of the "toe-up" foot activates the Chiao Mai Channels, thus encouraging energy flow to the brain. By co-ordinating the breath with the steps, the Fire and Water of the body will be mixed, automatically activating the Two Side Channels and the Central Channel and also the Little Earth.

STRATEGY NOTE | *It is interesting to note that both of the above exercises accomplish the same energizing of the brain, the first by pumping the arms and the second by pumping the legs.*

3.3 | SAI PING MA

THIS EXERCISE entails standing for two to five minutes in the familiar "legs bent, arms circled in front of chest" posture. The deeper the knees bend with keeping the spine straight, of course, the more effective the exercise (and more painful).

To get a good grasp of the strategy of this exercise, it is helpful to look at the body position in relationship to an I Ching Hexagram.

Hexagrams are composed of six lines, each representing either Yin or Yang depending on the energy associated with its position.

In the human body, the lines are represented by body areas as follows:

Line 1 | **Feet**
Line 2 | **Legs and Lower Back**
Line 3 | **Hypogastrium/Lower Burner**
Line 4 | **Epigastrium/Middle Burner**
Line 5 | **Chest/Upper Burner**
Line 6 | **Above the Neck**

Generally speaking, the lower body (below the waist) is considered Yin and the upper body (above the waist) is considered Yang. Lets take a closer look at the areas in question:

Line 1 | **Feet**
The bottom of the feet are the site of the acupuncture point Kidney 1, called 'Gushing Spring.' Located at the juncture of the anterior and middle third of the sole of the foot, 'Gushing Spring' is the point that connects Man to the Earth. When the Kidney 1 points on both feet are in contact with the Earth (as in **Sai Ping Ma**) the feet are in a Yin position. However; if one or both points are not touching the ground, the relative quality of the feet is Yang.

Line 2 | **Legs and Lower Back**
The closer to the Earth and the more static the legs are, the more Yin is their nature. When the legs are straight, they tend to move Chi up in the body thus emphasizing Yang qualities. When the knees are bent (as in **Sai Ping Ma**) the Chi sinks down towards the Earth emphasizing Yin qualities.

Line 3 | **Hypogastrium/Lower Burner**
The Lower Burner is close to the point where Yin changes to

Yang. It is the least Yin in the Yin area of the body. Movement will tend to encourage Yang qualities in this area, but in **Sai Ping Ma** the area is still.

Line 4 | **Epigastrium/Middle Burner**
Here again we have an area on the border of Yin and Yang. Without any alterations (as in **Sai Ping Ma**), the area is Yang.

Line 5 | **Chest/Upper Burner**
The chest is well into the Yang area of the body but in Chi Kung theory, the middle of the palms represent the Heart and Chest. If the hands are hanging at the sides, they can change the nature of the chest to Yin. In **Sai Ping Ma**, the hands and arms are held at Heart level thus maintaining the Yang nature of the chest.

Line 6 | **Head**
The head in its upright position (as in **Sai Ping Ma**) is Yang. The position of a man standing in **Sai Ping Ma** is represented by the hexagram:

The upper three lines (Yang) are the trigram representing Heaven and the lower three lines (Yin) are the trigram representing Earth. Thus, a man standing with legs apart and knees bent with his arms circled in front of his chest would be in a posture reflecting the natural Yin/Yang relationship of Heaven and Earth. This posture is commonly used by Chi Kung practitioners to align their energies with the natural flow of Chi in the universe.

Generally, this hexagram is not a fortunate symbol. With Heaven's energy rising and Earth's energy sinking, we find a situation where Yin and Yang are moving away from each other.

From a Chi Kung standpoint, there is one more piece in the picture—Man.

Man stands between Heaven and Earth, being formed by their interaction. By assuming a position of Yang energy (Heaven) on top and Yin energy (Earth) on the bottom and providing for their union by circulating his own Chi through the mechanism of breath, man can assist in the joining of the energies of Heaven and Earth in himself and reap substantial energetic rewards from his immersion in the natural flow of the universe.

There is always some part of Yin in Yang and some Yang in Yin. Heaven and Earth are the extremes of Yin and Yang in the universe. In nature, circulation between Heaven and Earth takes place by the Yin-Water in Heaven falling to nourish Earth as rain and the Yang-Fire in Earth rising from the molten core of the planet. Man, in the **Sai Ping Ma** position, facilitates that energetic interaction within himself and enjoys the fruits of the union.

Normally, Yin energy sinks and Yang energy rises, so it would appear that the energies of Heaven and Earth would not join internally in **Sai Ping Ma**. The catalyst for the inner circulation of those energies in Man is the breath. The rising and falling of the breath (through deep abdominal breathing) initiates the movement necessary to allow the interpenetration of Yin and Yang (Heaven and Earth) in Man.

3.4 | LADY RAISES LOTUS TO THE TEMPLE

THE LOTUS represents the product of refined Jing, Chi and Shen interpenetration, a relatively Yang substance. The Temple represents the Divine. The offering is made through the body, a Yin substance, represented by the Lady.

This exercise is a fairly simple yet profound set of movements performed much like Tai Chi Chuan (with only 8 movements). Its purpose is to gather and mix the 'Three Treasures' while simultaneously opening the practitioner to 'Universal Presence.'

STRATEGY NOTE | *In the previous two exercises, the system allows Universal Presence to manifest passively by* *presenting a physical form (**Sai Ping Ma**) to energetically match the universe and seeks Universal Presence through active physical and energetic manipulations (Lady Raises the Lotus to the Temple).*

3.5 | ENERGY TO THE FIRST TAN TIEN

THE FIRST TAN TIEN (Sky Eye, Third Eye, Ajna, House of Intelligence, Brow Center, Sixth Chakra etc.) is an area many disciplines seek to develop. This exercise is basically one way of working on that development.

The Ajna or Brow Center, is located between the eyebrows at the level of the medulla plexus and the pineal plexus. Also known as the Third Eye, it is the organ of clairvoyance symbolizing both the basic Yin/Yang polarity of the body and the concept of non-duality. The element of the Sixth Chakra is the pure essence of all the other elements, its color is transparent, luminescent bluish or camphor white and its planes are austerity and penance.

The Ajna Center is the seat of psychic powers, higher intuition and the mind/soul. This Chakra commands and controls the lower self.

Meditation on this center can eradicate all sins and impurities, bring knowledge of past lives and the future, and place the adept beyond all desires with no danger of backsliding. The adept will be able to control breath and mind, generate scriptures, and understand the inner meaning of cosmic knowledge. The Divine within will be revealed and the Divine in others reflected.

Congested energy in this Chakra may lead to egotistical and maniacally authoritative behavior, while weakness may lead to over sensitivity and lack of discipline.

The Pituitary Gland is associated with the Ajna Center, sometimes called 'the conductor of the endocrine orchestra.' The acupuncture point associated with this center is Yin Tang. The Pituitary Gland lies at the base of the brain behind the root of the nose. It is comprised of two distinct parts or lobes, the anterior lobe and the posterior lobe. Each lobe has its own embryological origin, history, functions and secretions in a somewhat Yin/Yang-Male/Female relationship with its other part.

The Anterior Pituitary originates in the mouth area and is the master of the whole endocrine system. Secretions of the anterior lobe stimulate growth of bone and connective tissue and stimulate the adrenal cortex, thyroid, and production of breast milk. They also influence pigment production in the skin. The anterior lobe helps balance the creative and sexual forces and skeletal growth.

"The Posterior Pituitary developed from the oldest part of the nervous system. Here, as in the Hypothalamus, we have a meeting of the endocrine and nervous systems. The Posterior Pituitary secretes hormones which control the salt and water content of the blood, raise blood pressure and stimulate plain muscle as in the uterus, gall bladder, ureter and urinary bladder. It also controls kidney secretions, and the sugar content of both blood and urine. Sleep cycles, intellectual growth and moral sense are influenced by the Pituitary." —*Magnetic Healing and Meditation* published by White Elephant Monastery

It is development of the First Tan Tien that allows people to see "auras" and also view their "inner landscape," which becomes very interesting with progress in Taoist Chi Kung. In later stages of training, just viewing certain "internal landscapes" is a valid training technique. This center is also used to communicate with the energies of nature.

The First Tan Tien is the center of consciousness. It is the 'command center' for all the bodily systems and states of awareness. Activation of this center is said to turn off the external mind and awaken inner awareness.

3.6 | HEAVEN AND EARTH STANDING

HEAVEN AND EARTH Standing is a technique that enables the practitioner to lead energy out the top of the head and the bottom of the feet to commune with the natural energies of Heaven and Earth. This is accomplished through filling the body with "breath," tightening the muscles and leading the energy with the mind which encourages the "full" energy to extrude through the appropriate openings. At advanced levels of training, the practitioner will often feel his energy spontaneously communicate and harmonize with Heaven and Earth energies at any time, regardless of the activity.

STRATEGY NOTE | *Again we have a pair of exercises that accomplish the same purpose utilizing opposite techniques (in regards to the polar opposites—Yin and Yang). Exercises 3.1 and 3.2 (pg. 151) used top and bottom. Exercises 3.3 (pg. 151) and 3.4 (pg. 154) utilized active and passive, while Exercises 3.5 (pg. 155) and 3.6 (pg. 156), utilized mind and body to open the practitioner to universal potentials.*

3.7 | WALKING ENERGY AND MIND TO FEET

THIS EXERCISE brings both physical and mental attention to the feet. As we have seen in previous exercises, the feet are extremely important to the balanced practice of Chi Kung. KI 1, the first point of the Kidney channel and the main point of interconnection between Earth and Man is on the bottom of the foot. Both Yin and Yang Chiao Mai *(see Yin/Yang Heel Pulse, exercise 2.36, pg. 145)* begin on the heel and the masterpoint of the Chong Mai or Central Channel *(see Energy to Chong Mai, exercise 2.5, pg. 112)* is on the side of the arch of the foot.

Balance is extremely important in any energetic practice, and especially so in practices that actually include transformative techniques. Although Level 3 is the "Spirit" Level of training, the exercises must take into consideration both the need to harmonize the upper and lower parts of the body and to link Heaven and Earth through Man. All too often incomplete practices emphasize the "up" techniques while neglecting the "down" side. Calamity is sure to follow.

Walking Energy and Mind to Feet utilizes the Yin/Yang shifting of energy caused by walking to accomplish both the engorging of the feet (alternately) with energy and to activate the Two Side Channels. The walking is done on the tiptoes to powerfully activate KI 1. The mind and energy are kept below the waist to bring "refined" energy downwards and link the Jing, Chi, and Shen (the "Flower").

STRATEGY NOTE | *This exercise is a set-up for the following one where the three parts of the "Flower" are not only linked and moved within the Central Channel but also brought to communicate with Heaven and, Earth.*

3.8 | RAISING THE FLOWER, LOWERING THE FLOWER

RAISING THE FLOWER, Lowering the Flower, as stated above, moves the interpenetrated Three Treasures up and down the Central Channel and extends that consciousness both up to Heaven and down into the Earth.

The exercise is one of the most demanding dynamic exercises in the system, involving full up and down movements with tension, three inhales without exhaling and a high level of energetic awareness.

STRATEGY NOTE | *After the powerful energetic experience of the previous exercise it is essential to provide a safety net to balance the body/mind/spirit, which is provided by the next exercise. Although an expert practitioner can perform any exercise in a balanced manner and rebalance himself with the usual Basic, it is prudent for beginners and experts alike to utilize all the safety mechanisms built into this system.*

3.9 | BALANCE BLOOD AND ENERGY IN THE BODY

AS AN EXERCISE to balance the flows of blood and energy in the body, Balance Blood and Energy in the Body is both simple and powerful.

After Gathering Energy in the Lower Tan Tien, the practitioner assumes the push-up position. He then performs six repetitions of "inside breathing" between his upper back and Lower Tan Tien. This both mixes the Fire and Water to "refine energy" and creates equal pressure throughout the body as the four limbs all bear approximately the same amount of weight.

The exercise ends with a Basic.

3.10 | POWER TO THE HANDS

THIS EXERCISE brings energetic attention to the Heart and Lungs (the Middle Tan Tien—CV 17). After balancing the blood and energy in the previous exercise, Power to the Hands energizes that area which controls most of the rhythms of all the circulation in the body.

The exercise involves Gathering Energy into the Lower Tan Tien, then extending and retracting the upper limbs twice while continuously inhaling. The movements plus the proper hand positions engorge the areas involved.

STRATEGY NOTE | *The previous two exercises are used to balance the flows and regulate the rhythms of Blood and Energy in the body.*

3.11 | KNEE SLEEPING

KNEE SLEEPING is an extremely powerful technique somewhat analogous to Maha Bandha in Yoga. If you review the material on Bandhas in the beginning of this book, you will see the three Bandhas mentioned.

Moola Bandha is used to seal the lower portion of the energy pathways in the spinal column and Jalandhara Bandha is used to seal the top portion of the energy pathways in the spinal column. In a way, this turns the spinal column into a "tube" with both ends capped. Uddiyana Bandha is used to increase the pressure in this "tube." The simultaneous practice of all three of these Bandhas is called Maha Bandha.

When Maha Bandha is released, the pressurized energy in the "tube" rushes throughout the body, toning, relaxing and rejuvenating the entire system.

This technique potentially energizes the deepest levels of the Central Channel, completely absorbs the individual in Cosmic Consciousness and unifies every aspect of being.

Knee Sleeping is performed by Gathering energy in the Lower Tan Tien and assuming a position on the floor where the body is balanced on the top of the head (Jalandhara Bandha) and the knees (slightly contracting the perineal muscles creates Moola Bhanda). Appropriate inside breathing techniques are then performed (Uddiyana Bandha). The practitioner may then stand and do a Basic or hold the position up to two minutes before doing the Basic.

3.12 | CONCENTRATION IN FOOT

AGAIN we have an exercise to activate the important channels relating to the foot and balance any disharmonious uprising energy in the body. This exercise differs from Walking Mind and Energy to the Feet in that it is stationary. Actually, Concentration in the Foot is extremely difficult to perform. The body will be balanced on one leg with the hands behind the back, the head down and the eyes closed. To maintain that position requires great concentration in the foot which of course brings energy and consciousness to that area.

Another benefit of exercises that bring attention to the feet is that they "clear the mind." The mind is considered Fire and the feet Water. By bringing the Fire to the Water, the mind is cleared (cooled) of negativity. Exercises like Concentration in the Foot, which are difficult to perform, increase the minds' ability to become "one pointed." Many systems consider that attaining this "one pointed" quality is an important step in the process of integrating the individual with the Divine.

STRATEGY NOTE | *A quick review of Walking Energy and Mind to the Feet will show us that after performing a foot exercise we followed with a moving energy up and down type exercise. In that case, moving the energy in the Central Channel. The same strategy appears here. After performing Concentration in Foot, we follow with Monkey Walking, an exercise that moves energy up and down in the Two Side Channels.*

3.13 | MONKEY WALKING

MONKEY WALKING generates great power in the body by alternately engorging each of the Two Side Channels with energy. It also mixes the Fire and Water, activates the Kidneys and opens the energetic pathways to the bones. The exercise is designed to bring energy up from Earth and down from Heaven and lead those energies to the deepest levels of the body.

This exercise is performed by Gathering Energy into the Lower Tan Tien and "walking" nine steps while raising the same side leg and arm and inhaling with each step. This motion activates KI 1, UB 11, GV 14, and GB 21.

"As we have already mentioned, GV 14 is the meeting place of all six Yang vessels of the hand and the six Yang vessels of the foot. As external diseases penetrate from the outside (Yang) towards the inside, this point is well suited to address external problems. GV 14 is not only able to expel external pathogens, but also able to tonify our defensive energy. Owing to its ability to control the pores, dispel pathogenic heat, and tonify deficiency, GV 14 is a major point in regulating the body's sweating. As one of the points directly relating to the Sea of Chi, GV 14 can also treat deficiency

and exhaustion of the whole body and painful obstructions anywhere in the body. GV 14 also affects the whole spinal column."
— *Level 1 | see pg. 65*

UB 11 is also a point that is very influential in activating the
defense mechanisms of the body. It is the "meeting place of the
bones" and is used to address any problems with the bones. As the
Kidneys "control the bones," UB 11 is closely associated with the
Kidneys. Our system of Chi Kung makes extensive use of this connection to the Kidneys and bones (especially the spine) in several
exercises.

UB 11 is also directly related to the "Sea of Blood." Chong Mai is
referred to as the Sea of Blood and UB 11 accesses that "Sea." This
point can increase blood flow, thus distributing essence. In high
level Chi Kung, Chong Mai is extensively used for transporting
refined energy to feed the Spirit.

"KI 1, referred to as 'Gushing Spring' (or Earth Surge) is the place
where the energies of Earth and Man conjoin. It is an important
point in balancing the body and absorbing energy from the Earth
to supplement the body's own energy."—*see pg. 152*

"GB 21 is an important point in directing Qi downwards in the
body. In fact, its downward function is so great that some systems use the point to collect Qi from Heaven." —*18 Buddha Hands
Qigong (Chi Kung)* published by White Elephant Monastery

The exercise ends with a Basic.

STRATEGY NOTE | *Leading energy to the bones is considered
one of the highest levels of Chi Kung practice. As the student
progresses, the bones will naturally develop increased ability to
interact with the body and the universe. Often, upper level Chi
Kung exercises are designed to speed up this process.*

Exercises which increase energy flow to the bones help to remove fat from the marrow, creating more space for marrow itself.
Marrow in round bones produces red blood cells (oxygenation of

the body) and marrow in flat bones produces white blood cells (immune system).

Bone exercises also strengthen the bone matrix which both stores energy and strengthens the bones. Energy absorbed from "bone breathing" strengthens the whole system. It is interesting to note that bones are crystalline in nature. This opens the door to many possibilities in the realm of energy and information storage.

3.14 | BLOOD AND ENERGY IN HAND

THIS SIMPLE EXERCISE utilizes intense arm swinging to engorge the hands with blood and energy. On the surface, it is an exercise that merely activates the channels that flow to and from the hands and of course, stimulates P 8, the energy "gate" in the palm. The purpose of this excrcise is much more far reaching than it appears.

The Heart is the link between our emotional nature and our Divine nature. The Spirits, emissaries of 'Heaven's Mandate,' reside in the Heart. At the same time, the Heart (through the "Radiant Spirits') governs the activities of the body, including physical, mental and emotional activities. If the activities governed by the Heart, "feedback" to the Heart in the form of desires, attachments, expectations, etc., the Heart becomes full in a negative sense. This explains the constant positive references to an "Empty Heart" found in ancient texts relating to spiritual progress.

The energy propels blood, rich in essences that hold Spirit, to link the Heart with the rest of the body. By physically moving blood and energy out of the Heart to the hands, this exercise "empties" the Heart to allow room for more 'Radiant Spirits' from Heaven to express themselves in Man.

3.15 | ENLARGE THE HEART PULSE

ENLARGE THE HEART PULSE utilizes breath and body position to encourage the "filling of the Heart (by 'Radiant

Spirits') and the grounding of those Spirits in Essence (by linking Heart and Kidneys). In other words, it encourages our reception to 'Heaven's Mandate.'

3.16 | ENERGY TO DU

DU refers to the Governing Vessel. This exercise specifically activates the beginning point of that Vessel, GV 1. In Yoga, this is the area activated by Moola Bandha.

In Taoist religious theory, 'Heaven's Mandate' is drawn into Man through the Heart, roots in Essence through the Kidneys, and rises up the spine to express itself in our individual lives through the Governing Vessel. According to how well we follow 'Heaven's Mandate,' as the Spirits rise up through the spine our "Karma" (lessons we need to learn in this life) is neutralized.

The goals of Chi Kung and many other spiritual practices are to maintain our health and increase the efficiency of the Karmic transformations so that all the lessons are learned and we can return to "Spirit."

Health is maintained through Level 1 practices dealing with Essence (balancing our form and the energies that support it). Level 2 exercises balance and bring together the opposite polarities of our being. This creates tremendous potential power that can reflect in Level 1 for our health and in Level 3 where it catalyses energy that transforms into a vehicle for consciousness to expand beyond the mundane realms of everyday life to the 'singularity of Divinity.'

Du or the Governing Vessel is one of the pathways through which transformation takes place and Du 1 (activated in this exercise) is the opening to that pathway as well as the inner spinal pathways of the Conception Vessel and Central Channel or Chong Mai.

Energy to Du has far reaching effects on the body/mind/spirit complex. Activating this area encourages the spontaneous alignment of the physical, mental and psychic energies. It regulates the internal organs by stimulating the nerves in the lower pelvic region and helps maintain hormone balance. By opening the spinal pathways, this exercise prepares one for 'spiritual awakening.'

The exercise is rather simple. It involves activating the area by posture and physical contraction of the muscles of the perineum while performing a long slow inhale. The exercise ends with a Basic.

STRATEGY NOTE | *Concerning the last three exercises, we have prepared the Heart to receive Spirit, opened the Heart to that reception and brought Spirit to Essence, Fire to Water, and concentrated that "mixture" at the gateway to the spinal pathways.*

From here, in the next three exercises we will totally open and connect the Three Tan Tiens through the spinal pathways, open and harmonize the Two Side Channels, and extrude the energy beyond the body.

3.17 | INSIDE LOOKING

INSIDE LOOKING is an exercise similar to Knee Sleeping in that the position used naturally fits the requirements for performing Maha Bandha. In this case, the practitioner is seated in a position reminiscent of Chong Mai *(see Energy to Chong Mai, exercise 2.5, pg. 112)*. Rather than use Uddiyana Bandha as the "force multiplier" for energy in the Central Channel, Inside Looking uses the mind, breath control and "inner sight" to activate the Heart (Middle Tan Tien) and then link the Heart to the Lower Tan Tien and the Upper Tan Tien. The exercise takes about seven minutes to complete and ends with a Basic.

3.18 | SHOULDER TWO

SHOULDER 2 is a walking exercise that activates and harmonizes the Two Side Channels and upper back and shoulders to lead transformed energy up through the spine to the head. It involves nine steps, nine inhales and ends with a Basic.

STRATEGY NOTE | *The above two exercises open the spinal pathways, one sitting exercise emphasizing mind regulation and one moving exercise emphasizing body regulation—both with breath regulation.*

3.19 | OUTSIDE LOOKING

OUTSIDE LOOKING is a simple sitting exercise that links the Lower Tan Tien to the external environment through mind regulation and "sight." It is a precursor to more advanced energy gathering practices

3.20 | LIFE TO CHONG MAI

This is a very powerful exercise using "inside breathing" and a shoulder stand to totally engorge the Chong Mai (Central Channel) with energy.

3.21 | ENERGY AND BLOOD TO EYES

ENERGY AND BLOOD to Eyes does in fact bring those two substances to the eyes. Although the correct posture and breath control aids in this result, the intense concentration needed to perform the exercise and the pathways activated causes an energetic engorgement of the Upper Tan Tien—Spirit House. Blood and Energy also represent the basic Yin and Yang of the body. This exercise brings the opposites together in the Upper Tan Tien, which is the fundamental prerequisite for nourishing the Spirit. Using various eye movement and control techniques is common in high level Taoist Chi Kung

STRATEGY NOTE | *In the previous two exercises we have opened the Central Channel and brought the basic Yin and Yang of the body together and concentrated that union in the Upper Tan Tien, the center of consciousness. The next step in spiritual transformation is to link the individual consciousness to the Universal Consciousness (see Open the Top, exercise, 3.22 below).*

In theory, this process neutralizes all past karma, vastly expands intuitive knowledge, and brings the consciousness to the fourth dimension and beyond

3.22 | OPEN THE TOP

OPEN THE TOP is an exercise that seeks to draw Heavenly Energy through the top of the head to the Lower Tan Tien. Aside from the body nourishing benefits of this energy (gathering Energy from Heaven), the consciousness expanding benefits are enormous.

3.23 | EAR TWO

EAR TWO utilizes breath control and the mind to engorge each of the Two Side Channels with energy. In a way, it is like a Blood and Energy to the Eyes for the ears. The second half of the exercise utilizes "tapping" on the back of the head to consolidate the Spirit.

3.24 | YIN/YANG, LEFT/RIGHT BREATHING

THIS EXERCISE involves tensing one side of the body at a time to engorge the Two Side Channels specifically and the two sides of the body in general.

STRATEGY NOTE | *The previous two exercises use a sitting "mind" practice and a standing "body" practice to activate and harmonize the Two Side Channels. The obvious next step is to open the Central Channel as in Energy from Tan Tien to Head.*

3.25 | ENERGY FROM TAN TIEN TO HEAD (EAGLE)

THIS EXERCISE is an extremely powerful technique for opening the Central Channel. Utilizing strong body and arm movements that activate the Two Side Channels, dynamic internal breath control and intense concentration, the Eagle vigorously opens the Central Channel.

3.26 | STOMACH AND INTESTINES
TO UPPER BACK

LIKE THE EAGLE, Stomach and Intestines to Upper Back brings energy up the spine to the head. In this case the Two Side Channels are activated by a walking pattern while the energy is led up the Central Channel by body position, breath and mind.

The exercise gets its name from the powerful activation of the rising fire of the Ming Men, one of whose functions is to support the energy that keeps the organs in place in the body.

STRATEGY NOTE | *Each of the two previous exercises activates the Two Side Channels and moves energy up the Central Channel. The Eagle accents arm movements to accomplish this and Stomach and Intestines to Upper Back accents leg movements.*

3.27 | CLOSE THE NINE HOLES

CLOSE THE NINE HOLES is a technique to withdraw sense perception and eliminate mental processes. The Nine Holes are the two eyes, two ears, two nostrils, mouth, and the two lower orifices. The energies from these nine openings are withdrawn to the Lower Tan Tien until consciousness alone remains. Control of these energies is said to "stop the mind," eliminating all thoughts, emotions, and desires which are modifications of the Original Mind. Individual consciousness is replaced with Universal Consciousness.

Advanced practitioners can reach a state beyond duality where only the experience exists. This state beyond time and space is referred to as 'Enlightenment.'

When the mind stops, breath also spontaneously stops. This is a precursor to advanced "Hibernating Breathing" techniques.

3.28 | LOWER BLOOD PRESSURE

LOWERING BLOOD PRESSURE is another "safety valve" exercise. It directs energy and consciousness to the feet to use Earth energy to balance any upward disharmony in the body.

3.29 | SUN DING FUT

SUN DING FUT is the state of absolute singularity. Basically, the practitioner attains the state of Close the Nine Holes and then gives up the attachment to that experience to reach—Tao. At this point, the practitioner ceases to exist as a separate entity.

This state is sometimes called "Hibernation" in Chi Kung circles. When the breath and mind are suspended for long periods of time, the animal functions slow down to the least activity necessary to sustain the body. When the conditioned mind and animal functions "hibernate" the individual modifications of mind and energy diminish and the practitioner becomes harmonized with Singularity, the Universal Principle or Tao.

3.30 | SPIRIT OUT

THIS IS AN EXERCISE for developing the Spirit's ability to expand beyond the body. Aside from the obvious advantages such an expansion would bring to ones "small view of life," the Spirit returns with "Essences" that nourish the being. An accomplished practitioner can travel anywhere in the universe with full consciousness.

A human being is capable of projecting energy/consciousness outside of his physical form, releasing that energy/consciousness from the limitations of the form. This "field" of conscious/energy can be controlled, taking on any spatial dimension and geographical location desired. At high levels of development, this "field" can have practical applications. When dealing with the interactions between and combinations of the consciousness inside and outside the body, an unlimited variety of "conscious/energy" fields are possible.

THIS EXERCISE is an extreme version of Chong Mai (from Level 2, pg. 112). After Gathering Energy in the Lower Tan Tien, the rest of the exercise is all done with "inside breathing." Extra power is developed through the use of a belt around the waist.

In most systems of Chi Kung, loose clothing is recommended to allow a smooth, free flow of energy. In our system, a belt is used to accent the Tan Tien area and in this case to add power to the exercise.

The exercise does develop the Tan Tien and the Ming Men. As in Chong Mai *(see Energy to Chong Mai, exercise 2.5, pg. 112)* it also has the ability to correct any deviations in the Central Channel, which is essential to the safety of the practitioner.

The alternate name "Put Out Fat" is used to describe the effect of a developed Tan Tien and an opened Central Channel on the practitioner. Fat is a stagnation. If there is fat on the exterior body, there will be fat inside also, retarding circulation in the organs. At a high level of development, when powerful refined energies are circulating throughout the body, stagnation is dangerous. When the fire of Ming Men is well developed and co-penetrating the Tan Tien, the metabolism will naturally both burn off excess fat and balance desires for food that would lead to excess fat storage.

The Central Channel also plays a role in weight management. As we age, production of human growth hormone diminishes. Produced in the anterior pituitary gland, one of the functions of this gland is to regulate the composition (fat/lean muscle) of the body. A decline in human growth hormone initiates a decline in lean muscle and an increase in fat.

The Central Channel brings "refined energy/consciousness" to the brain. This includes energizing the glands in that area. By keeping the anterior pituitary gland vitalized through a well developed, functioning Central Channel, the decline in human growth hormone will be greatly reduced. This, of course, will reduce the amount of fat stored in the body.

One problem with modern times is the amount of calorie rich foods available to the practitioner. This was not true of ancient times, especially of practitioners living in "wild" places close to nature. By the nature of the food available today we face dietary problems that are different than those faced by the originators of our system. We have to rely on both the balancing functions of the practices and our own intelligence to make sane choices about our eating habits. In theory, proper development will bring us the understanding and the will to support our practices with proper diet.

The diet guidelines for our system are "eat all you want" for the first twenty years or so and, thereafter, slowly begin to reduce food intake with occasional fasting. The fasting is not just refraining from eating but "living on Essence" which is gathering Essences from nature to support the physical form. Again, these guidelines must be tempered by the times.

3.32 | CONTROL SPIRIT

CONTROL SPIRIT is an intense concentration of energy in the Spirit House. The Upper Tan Tien-Spirit House has been well described previously.

STRATEGY NOTE | *Control Spirit becomes even more intense after performing Put Out Fat which gets the Transformational Fires blazing and opens the Central Channel. That "Controlled Spirit" is fully utilized in the next exercise.*

3.33 | INSPECT OUTSIDE

INSPECT OUTSIDE is a high level exercise that is used to expand the consciousness beyond the confines of the body. It combines Close the Nine Holes, Energy to the First Tan Tien and Spirit Out.

3.34 | FIRE IN THE TAN TIEN

FIRE IN THE TAN TIEN utilizes breath control and a turning of the head from side to side to activate the Ming Men/Two Side Channels and the Belt Channel. The Original Fire of Ming Men is stimulated and led to the Tan Tien, both from the inside directly and through the Belt Channel indirectly.

3.35 | BONES

THIS IS A straightforward exercise aimed at directing energy deep into the bones through activation of the Two Side Channels/Ming Men and UB 11—'master point of the bones.'

3.36 | BIG EARTH

IN MOST SYSTEMS of Taoist Chi Kung, Big Earth is an advanced technique that involves circulating energy through all of the Eight Extra-Ordinary Vessels as opposed to Little Earth which just circulates energy through the Conception and Governing Vessels.

In Hua Shan Taoist Chi Kung, Big Earth involves engorging the entire body with energy while concentrating on the tip of the nose and inhaling. As we stated before, the tip of the nose was thought to be the first materialization of the Ming Men energy, linking the physical form to the original meeting of Jing, Chi and Shen. Thus, our Big Earth brings the individual's energy to singularity and joins that to the place of 'energetic conception.'

STRATEGY NOTE | *The Big Earth technique is supported by both activating the Ming Men/Tan Tien through Fire in the Tan Tien and activating the deepest energies in the body through Bones.*

In Conclusion

THIS COMPLETES the foundation of Hua Shan Taoist Chi Kung. All the necessary principles and techniques for total energetic/spiritual development are contained in these 108 positions. Although these exercises can be learned in a relatively short amount of time, it takes decades of devoted study to master them and reap the full benefits available from the system.

There are a number of other exercises in the system. Some of them are taught to students at particular times for developmental reasons. Many of them are just different ways of doing things already covered in the "foundation." No practitioner has time to do all the exercises. Since each practitioner is an individual, he will gravitate to certain exercises depending on his own level of development and consciousness. Ample opportunity is presented to the student to manifest his own individuality through the system.

In closing, I would like to thank my teacher, Chan Chiu Lim, for his patience, understanding and generosity in teaching me.
I would also like to thank my own students for their support and interest in preserving this treasure from the past.

Good Training!

—LARRY JOHNSON | O.M.D., L. Ac.

APPENDIX

(Acupuncture points mentioned in the text)

GV 4 | Ming Men | Located on the midline of the back below the spinous process of the second lumbar vertebra. Tonifies the Kidneys, Essence and Source Chi—regulates the water passages—benefits the bones and low back—drains dampness—regulates the Governing Vessel

GV 9 | Supreme Yang | Located on the midline of the back below the spinous process of the seventh thoracic vertebra. Strengthens the Spleen—regulates the Liver and Gall Bladder—clears Liver Fire—transforms damp/heat—regulates the Middle Burner

GV 14 | Big Vertebra | Located on the midline of the back below the spinous process of the seventh cervical vertebra. Calms the Spirit and clears the brain—tonifies protective Chi—dispels Wind and Wind Heat—tonifies deficiency—relaxes the sinews—clears Fire, Heat, and Summer heat—firms the exterior

GV 16 | Palace of Wind | Located on the midline of the neck just below the occipital protuberance. Eliminates Wind, Wind/Cold and Wind/Heat—nourishes the Sea of Marrow—opens the sensory orifices

GV 20 | Hundred Meetings | Located on the midline of the head at the vertex. Pacifies wind and subdues Yang—calms the Spirit—clears the brain—spreads Liver Chi—revives consciousness

CV 12 | Middle Cavity | Located on the midline of the abdomen halfway between the umbilicus and the sternocostal angle. Harmonizes the Middle Burner and subdues rebellion—strengthens the Stomach and Spleen—reduces digestive stagnation—regulates Chi and Blood—transforms damp

LU 1 | Middle Palace | Located six body inches from the midline of the chest below the acromonial extremity of the clavicle one body inch below the infraclavicular fossa. Regulates the Lungs and Upper Burner tonifies the Lungs—transforms phlegm, clears heat and regulates the water passages—tonifies Ancestral Chi

LU 2 | Cloud Gate | Located below the acromonial extremity of the clavicle in the depression lateral to the triangle of m. pectoralis, six body inches from the midline of the chest. Clears Lung Heat—descends Lung Chi—dispels fullness

ST 25 | Heaven's Pivot | Two Body inches lateral to the umbilicus. Regulates Chi, Blood, the intestines, Spleen, Stomach,Middle Burner and Lower Burner—resolves Dampness and Damp/Heat—reduces digestive stagnation

ST 36 | Leg Three Miles | Three Body inches below the knee and one fingerbreadth lateral to the anterior crest of the tibia. Clears fire and calms the Spirit—tonifies Chi and nourishes Blood and Yin-reduces digestive stagnation—resolves Dampness-tonifies the Kidneys and Lungs-regulates, strengthens and tonifies the Spleen—tonifies Source Chi, Chi and Blood—regulates and moistens the intestines—dispels Wind and Cold—revives Yang and restores consciousness

SP 21 | Great Envelope | Located in the sixth intercostal space on the mid-axillary line midway between the axilla and the free end of the eleventh rib—Regulates Chi and Blood—firms the sinews and joints facilitates Chi and Blood flow

UB 11 | Great Shuttle | Located one and one half body inches lateral to the lower border of the spinous process of the first thoracic vertebra–Benefits the bones and joints—expels pathogenic factors—regulates Lung Chi and alleviates cough

KI 1 | Gushing Spring | Located on the sole of the foot between the second and third metatarsal bones one third of the distance from the base of the second toe to the back of the heel. Tonifies the Kidneys and Essence—Calms the Spirit-revives consciousness—clears fire and heat—restores collapsed Yang—transforms Heart phlegm

TB 4 | Yang Pool | Located on the back of the hand at the level of the wrist between the tendons of extensor digitorum communis and extensor digiti minimi. Clears fire and Heat—dispels Wind—relaxes the sinews

GB 23 | Flank Sinews | Below the axilla in the fifth intercostal space at the level of the nipple—regulates Chi in the Three Burners—regulates the Liver, Gall Bladder, and Stomach—transforms Damp/Heat

GB 24 | Sun and Moon | Located directly below the nipple in the seventh intercostal space. Regulates the Liver, Gall Bladder, and Stomach—transforms Damp/Heat—harmonizes the Middle Burner

LIV 13 | Completion Gate | Located at the tip of the free end of the eleventh rib. Harmonizes the Liver and Spleen—regulates the Middle and Lower Burners—strengthens the Spleen—spreads Liver Chi—regulates Chi and Blood—transforms Dampness, Damp/Heat and Phlegm

LIV 14 | Cycle Gate | Located directly below the nipple in the sixth intercostal space. Spreads the Liver Chi—regulates the Liver and Gall Bladder—transforms Damp/Heat—harmonizes Liver and Stomach—invigorates Blood and softens masses ☯

BIBLIOGRAPHY

Chia, Mantak and Maneewan. *Awaken Healing Light of the Tao.* New York: Healing Tao Books/Huntington, 1993.

Deadman, Peter and Mazin, Al-Khafaji. *A Manual of Accupunture.* Hove, East Sussex, England: Journal of Chinese Medicine Publications, 1998

Johnson, Larry. *18 Buddha Hands Qigong (Chi Kung).* Crestone, Colorado: White Elephant Monastery, 1998

Johnson, Larry. *18 Buddha Hands Qigong (Chi Kung)—A Medical I Ching Exploration.* Crestone, Colorado: White Elephant Monastery, 1999

Lade, Arnie. *Images And Functions.* Seattle, Washington: Eastland Press, 1989.

Matsumoto, Kiiko and Birch, Stephen. *Hara Diagnosis: Reflections On The Sea.* Brookline, Massachusetts: Paradigm Publication, 1988.

ABOUT THE AUTHOR

LARRY JOHNSON'S study of Energetic Practices has spanned over 50 years. His work began with the study of Chinese Martial Arts and expanded to the fields of Oriental Medicine, Acupuncture, Chi Kung, Wu Style Tai Chi and Meditation.

Larry began his study of Hua Shan Taoist Chi Kung under Chan Chiu Lim in 1976 and became the only lineage disciple of Master Chan.

In 1978, Larry was given permission to teach Choy Lee Fut Kung Fu by Grandmaster Ming Jew.

In 1982 Larry passed the California State Examination for Licensed Acupuncturists. He received his Doctor of Oriental Medicine (O.M.D.) degree from the California Acupuncture College in 1983.

Larry has retired from teaching and continues to cultivate energetic refinement through his Chi Kung, Tai Chi, and Meditation practices.

BOOKS BY THE AUTHOR

Magnetic Healing and Meditation

Energetic Tai Chi Chuan

18 Buddha Hands Qigong

18 Buddha Hands Qigong • Instructional Video (DVD)

18 Buddha Hands Qigong • *A Medical I Ching Exploration*

Gemstone Prescriptions • *Handbook for Common Ailments*

Strategies • *Taoist Chi Kung* | Level 1

Strategies • *Taoist Chi Kung* | Levels 2 & 3

Yoga Meditation

Yoga Alchemy

Tai Chi Chuan Alchemy

Yoga Numerology

Strategies • *Taoist Chi Kung* | Levels 1, 2 & 3
THIRD EDITION 2026

TO ORDER

bfrank1394@protonmail.com

QUALIFIED HUA SHAN CHI KUNG TEACHERS

*Private instruction in Hua Shan Taoist Chi Kung
is available on an individual basis.*

CALIFORNIA

ANN | amquigley@me.com

ERIKA | erika@erikatrice.com

ROBIN | robinrosario@comcast.net

COLORADO

BUDDY | bfrank1394@protonmail.com

CHRISTIAN | christiandillo@gmail.com

JAMPAL | new108nomad@gmail.com

SUE | Knable.sue@gmail.com

www.ingramcontent.com/pod-product-compliance
Lightning Source LLC
Chambersburg PA
CBHW071515140726
47997CB00005B/1972